Environmental Health Criteria 122

n-HEXANE

Published under the joint sponsorship of
the United Nations Environment Programme,
the International Labour Organisation,
and the World Health Organization

First draft prepared by Dr K. Chipman,
University of Birmingham, United Kingdom

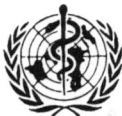

World Health Organization
Geneva, 1991

The **International Programme on Chemical Safety (IPCS)** is a joint venture of the United Nations Environment Programme, the International Labour Organisation, and the World Health Organization. The main objective of the IPCS is to carry out and disseminate evaluations of the effects of chemicals on human health and the quality of the environment. Supporting activities include the development of epidemiological, experimental laboratory, and risk-assessment methods that could produce internationally comparable results, and the development of manpower in the field of toxicology. Other activities carried out by the IPCS include the development of know-how for coping with chemical accidents, coordination of laboratory testing and epidemiological studies, and promotion of research on the mechanisms of the biological action of chemicals.

WHO Library Cataloguing in Publication Data

n-Hexane.

    (Environmental health criteria ; 122)

    1.Hexanes - adverse effects   2.Hexanes - toxicity   I.Series

    ISBN 92 4 157122 5   (NLM Classification: QV 633)
    ISSN 0250-863X

©World Health Organization 1991

PRINTED IN FINLAND
91/8768 — Vammala— 5000

CONTENTS

ENVIRONMENTAL HEALTH CRITERIA
FOR *n*-HEXANE

WHO TASK GROUP ON ENVIRONMENTAL HEALTH CRITERIA FOR n-HEXANE

Members

Professor E.A. Bababunmi, Department of Tropical Paediatrics, Liverpool School of Tropical Medicine, Liverpool, United Kingdom (*Rapporteur*)

Dr M. Cikrt, Centre of Industrial Hygiene and Occupational Diseases, Institute of Hygiene and Epidemiology, Prague, Czechoslovakia (*Vice-Chairman*)

Dr S. Dobson, Pollution and Ecotoxicology Section, Institute of Terrestrial Ecology, Monks Wood Experimental Station, Huntingdon, United Kingdom

Professor C.L. Galli, Toxicology Laboratory, Institute of Pharmacological Sciences, University of Milan, Milan, Italy (*Chairman*)

Dr S.D. Gangolli, British Industrial Biological Research Association, Carshalton, Surrey, United Kingdom

Dr C. Konantakieti, Technical Division, Food and Drug Administration, Ministry of Public Health, Bangkok, Thailand

Dr O. Ladefoged, Laboratory of Pathology, Institute of Toxicology, National Food Agency of Denmark, Ministry of Health, Soborg, Denmark

Professor A. Massoud, Department of Community Environmental and Occupational Medicine, Ainshams Faculty of Medicine, Cairo, Egypt

Dr V. Riihimäki, Department of Industrial Hygiene and Toxicology, Institute of Occupational Health, Helsinki, Finland

Observer

Dr H.P.A. Illing, Health and Safety Executive, Bootle, Merseyside, United Kingdom

Secretariat

Dr P.G. Jenkins, International Programme on Chemical Safety, World Health Organization, Geneva, Switzerland

Ms B. Labarthe, International Register of Potentially Toxic Chemicals, United Nations Environment Programme, Geneva, Switzerland

Dr E. Smith, International Programme on Chemical Safety, World Health Organization, Geneva, Switzerland (*Secretary*)

NOTE TO READERS OF THE CRITERIA DOCUMENTS

Every effort has been made to present information in the criteria monographs as accurately as possible without unduly delaying their publication. In the interest of all users of the environmental health criteria monographs, readers are kindly requested to communicate any errors that may have occurred to the Manager of the International Programme on Chemical Safety, World Health Organization, Geneva, Switzerland, in order that they may be included in corrigenda, which will appear in subsequent volumes.

*   *   *

A detailed data profile and a legal file can be obtained from the International Register of Potentially Toxic Chemicals, Palais des Nations, 1211 Geneva 10, Switzerland (Telephone No. 7988400 or 7985850).

ENVIRONMENTAL HEALTH CRITERIA FOR n-HEXANE

A WHO Task Group on Environmental Health Criteria for n-Hexane met in Carshalton, United Kingdom, from 12 to 16 March 1990. Dr E.M. Smith opened the meeting and welcomed the participants on behalf of the heads of the three IPCS cooperating organizations (UNEP/ILO/WHO). The Task Group reviewed and revised the draft criteria document and made an evaluation of the health risks of exposure to n-hexane.

The first draft of this document was prepared by Dr K. Chipman, University of Birmingham, United Kingdom. The second draft was also prepared by Dr Chipman, incorporating comments received following circulation of the first draft to IPCS contact points for Environmental Health Criteria monographs. Particularly valuable comments on the draft were made by the National Food Agency, Denmark, the National Institute of Public Health and Environmental Protection, The Netherlands, the European Chemical Industry Ecology and Toxicology Centre (ECETOC), and the US Environmental Protection Agency, National Institute of Environmental Health Sciences, Food and Drug Administration, and Centers for Disease Control.

Dr E.M. Smith and Dr P.G. Jenkins, both members of the IPCS Central Unit, were responsible for the overall scientific content and technical editing, respectively, of this monograph.

The efforts of all who helped in the preparation and finalization of the document are gratefully acknowledged.

* * *

Financial support for the Task Group was provided by the United Kingdom Department of Health as part of its contributions to IPCS. Partial financial support for the publication of this monograph was kindly provided by the United States Department of Health and Human Services, through a contract from the National Institute of Environmental Health Sciences, Research Triangle Park, North Carolina, USA - a WHO Collaborating Centre for Environmental Health Effects.

ABBREVIATIONS

ACGIH   American Conference of Government Industrial Hygienists

ADI   acceptable daily intake

BAER   brainstem auditory-evoked response

EEC   European Economic Community

EEG   electroencephalogram

EMG   electromyography

ip   intraperitoneal

MEK   methyl ethyl ketone

NOEL   no-observed-effect level

TWA   time-weighted average

1. SUMMARY

n-Hexane (normal hexane) is a colourless, volatile liquid. Commercial hexane is mainly a mixture of hexane isomers and related 6-carbon compounds, and has an *n*-hexane content varying between 20 and 80%. Gas chromatography coupled with flame ionization detection or mass spectroscopy is a suitable technique for the measurement of *n*-hexane. Occupational exposure limits range from 100-1800 mg/m^3 (time-weighted average, TWA) and 400-1500 mg/m^3 (ceiling value, CLV) in various countries.

n-Hexane can be isolated from natural gas and crude oil. It is used in food processing, including the extraction of vegetable oil, and as a solvent in various products and processes.

Once emitted into the environment, *n*-hexane exists predominantly in the vapour phase. In the atmosphere its half-life is estimated to be approximately 2 days, based on its reactivity with the OH radical alone. Reported LC_{50} values for aquatic organisms are few and variable and have been conducted under inappropriate conditions; an assessment of the toxic effects of *n*-hexane in this environment is, therefore, not possible. Low water solubility and high volatility make exposure of aquatic organisms unlikely except from uncontrolled discharge into surface waters.

In mammals, *n*-hexane is absorbed rapidly through the lungs and is distributed widely in the adult body, as well as to fetal tissue. Dermal absorption is limited. *n*-Hexane is metabolized oxidatively to a number of compounds, including 2,5-hexanedione, which is thought to be the ultimate neurotoxic agent. Particularly high levels of *n*-hexane and 2,5-hexanedione can occur in the sciatic nerve of rats. Most *n*-hexane is excreted unchanged in exhaled air; some is excreted as metabolites in exhaled air and urine.

n-Hexane is of low acute toxicity for adult rats by oral administration or inhalation. Oral LD_{50} values of 15-30 g/kg have been recorded, and an inhalation LC_{50}

value of 271 040 mg/m³ (77 000 ppm) has been reported for a 1-h exposure. At high vapour concentrations, animals show ataxia, seizures, and signs of central nervous system depression.

Testicular lesions and neurotoxicity appear to be the principal effects of repeated *n*-hexane exposure in rats. Severe testicular lesions have resulted from inhalation exposure to *n*-hexane and oral exposure to 2,5-hexanedione. Effects have been attributed to disruption of the cytoskeleton of Sertoli cells. There are secondary effects on post-spermatogonial germ cells, which disappear from affected tubules. Testicular effects were reversible after a single exposure for 24 h to 17 600 mg/m³ (5000 ppm) but irreversible after a 2-week exposure to the same concentration for 16 h/day, 6 days/week. 2,5-Hexanedione at 1% in drinking-water produced similar reversible testicular lesions after 2 to 3 weeks of dosing and irreversible effects (within 17 weeks) after 5 weeks of dosing.

The neurotoxic effect is characterized clinically by hind limb weakness, which can progress to paralysis. Axonal swellings develop in ' the central and peripheral nervous systems; more severe lesions (axonal degeneration and loss) can occur, particularly in the longest, largest-diameter nerves. In essentially continuous 6-month inhalation studies, peripheral and central nervous system lesions were present at doses of 1760 mg/m³ (500 ppm) or more, but no clinical or pathological effects were noted at 440 mg/m³ (125 ppm). Only limited recovery of amplitude of the fifth brainstem auditory-evoked response (believed to reflect central nervous system activity) and tail nerve action potential was recorded 15-22 weeks after cessation of continuous exposure to a vapour concentration of 3520 mg/m³ (1000 ppm), 5 days/week, for 11 weeks. Discontinuous exposure of rats to 3168 mg/m³ (900 ppm) for 72 weeks did not cause any apparent peripheral or central nervous system lesions, but there was some evidence of electrophysiological effects on peripheral nerves.

n-Hexane-induced neurotoxicity can be enhanced by combined exposure to methyl ethyl ketone, methyl isobutyl ketone, and lead acetate, and decreased by co-exposure to toluene. Toluene and *n*-hexane also have a synergistic effect in the disturbance of dopamine levels.

Severe microscopic lesions were noted in skin when *n*-hexane was applied dermally under occlusive conditions for short periods. Prolonged exposure to an *n*-hexane vapour concentration of 10 560 mg/m^3 (3000 ppm) can cause conjunctival irritation in rats and marked ocular irritation in rabbits. No skin sensitization data are available from animal studies.

Chromosomal damage (polyploidy in one study, structural aberrations in a second study) has been reported in both *in vitro* and *in vivo* studies. No increase in point mutation frequency or effects in tests for DNA damage has been noted.

There has been one carcinogenicity study with *n*-hexane (skin painting on mice), which provided no evidence of carcinogenicity.

The reproductive toxicity of *n*-hexane has not been studied adequately. There was no substantial evidence of embryotoxicity or teratogenicity in rats following inhalation, though concentrations were relatively low, or in mice after oral dosing. Postnatal development of rats was transiently delayed when dams were exposed to an *n*-hexane vapour concentration of 3520 mg/m^3 (1000 ppm).

Very little information is available on the acute toxicity of *n*-hexane to humans. Most studies have involved occupational exposure to solvent mixtures. The available data suggest that *n*-hexane has low acute toxicity. Signs of central nervous system depression, such as drowsiness, vertigo, and giddiness, have been reported after exposure to a commercial hexane level of 3520 to 17 600 mg/m^3 (1000-5000 ppm) for 10-60 min.

n-Hexane is a mild irritant causing transient erythema when in contact with human skin for short periods. More severe effects (erythema and blistering) were documented after occlusive skin contact for 5 h with commercial grade hexane. There have been no case reports of sensitization of skin in exposed workers, and no skin sensitization was noted in a maximization test with *n*-hexane.

On repeated exposure, *n*-hexane is neurotoxic, inducing a type of sensorimotor peripheral neuropathy. Many studies on the prevalence of *n*-hexane-induced neurotoxicity have been published; however, adequate exposure data are often lacking. Exposure to n-hexane concentrations in air varying from 106-8800 mg/m^3 (30-2500 ppm) has been associated with neuropathy. Cases of marked peripheral neuropathy were reported among Japanese sandal workers and Taiwanese press proofers exposed to n-hexane levels of approximately 176 and 352 mg/m^3 (50 and 100 ppm), respectively, for periods exceeding 8 h per day. In many cases exposure measurements were recent and probably did not accurately reflect previous exposures causing neuropathy.

Several cross-sectional studies have independently reported mild subclinical effects (for example, electrophysiological changes in peripheral nerves) in workers exposed to 70-352 mg/m^3 (20-100 ppm). However, no clear cases of clinically overt peripheral neuropathy were identified in any of these studies at exposure levels of less than 352 mg/m^3 (100 ppm).

The effects of n-hexane on the central nervous system have been investigated only in a few studies. Changes in somatosensory evoked potentials recorded from workers exposed to n-hexane were suggested to result from a central nerve conduction block. Altered visual evoked potentials and EEG traces have also been noted. These results suggest that n-hexane may produce central nervous system dysfunction, but the available data provide no information on related exposure levels.

2. IDENTITY, PHYSICAL AND CHEMICAL PROPERTIES, ANALYTICAL METHODS

2.1 Identity

Common synonyms: Hexyl hydride, hexane, Skellysolve B

Chemical structure:

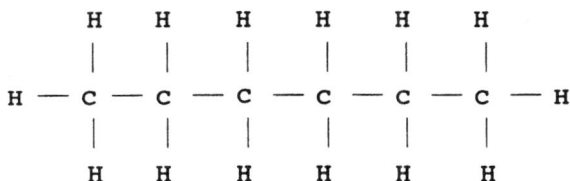

```
        H     H     H     H     H     H
        |     |     |     |     |     |
H  —  C  —  C  —  C  —  C  —  C  —  C  —  H
        |     |     |     |     |     |
        H     H     H     H     H     H
```

Chemical formula: C_6H_{14}

CAS registry number: 110-54-3

Relative molecular mass: 86.177

2.2 Physical and chemical properties

Some physical and chemical properties of various grades of *n*-hexane are given in Table 1.

n-Hexane is colourless, highly volatile (NIOSH, 1977a), and flammable (Dale & Drehman, 1980; ACGIH, 1986). It is poorly soluble in water but is soluble in most organic solvents including ethanol and ether (McAuliffe, 1963; NIOSH, 1977a; ACGIH, 1986).

Purified *n*-hexane contains 95-99.5% *n*-hexane, together with small amounts of other hexane isomers as impurities (Mellan, 1977; Baker & Rickert, 1981; Sandmeyer, 1981). Traces of benzene (0.05%) have been detected (Baker & Rickert, 1981). Commercial hexane is a mixture of hexane isomers (*n*-hexane, 2-methylpentane, 3-methylpentane, 2,3-dimethylbutane), cyclohexane, methyl cyclopentane and small amounts of pentane and heptane isomers, acetone,

Table 1. Physical and chemical properties of *n*-hexane[a]

Boiling point (°C)	68.74[b]
Melting point (°C)	-95.35[b]
Relative density (20 °C/4 °C)	0.66
Vapour pressure (25 °C)	20 kPa (150 mmHg)
Vapour density	2.97
Autoignition temperature (°C)	225
Explosive limit in air (% by volume)	1.1-7.5
Flash point (°C)	-21.7
Closed-cup flash point (°C)[c]	-30.56
Solubility in water (mg/litre at 25 °C)	9.5
Log *n*-octanol/water partition coefficient (log P_{ow} at 25 °C)	3.6
Refractive index (20 °C)	1.37
Colour, Saybolt	+39

[a] From: Mellan (1977)and IRPTC (1990).
[b] From: Clayton & Clayton (1981).
[c] From: ACGIH (1986).

methyl ethyl ketone, dichloromethane, and trichloroethyl-ene (Perbellini et al., 1981a,b,c; ACGIH, 1986). The *n*-hexane content of commercial hexane (Table 2) can vary between 20% and 80% (ACGIH, 1986).

Table 2. Composition (% by weight) of different grades of *n*-hexane[a]

	Research grade	Pure grade	Technical grade
n-Hexane	99.98	99.5	95-97.7
2-Methylpentane	trace	trace	trace
3-Methylpentane	0.02	0.1	0.2
Methylcyclopentane	trace	0.4	2.1

[a] From: Mellan (1977).

Pure *n*-hexane contains approximately 0.0005% of non-volatile material (Mellan, 1977), whereas commercial hexane may contain up to 0.04% (Patty & Yant, 1929; Vicedo et al., 1985). In commercial hexane, a number of phthalate esters (including dimethyl, diethyl, di-*n*-butyl, di-isobutyl, dihexyl, and diethylhexyl), adipate esters (dibutyl and dioctyl), and organophosphorus compounds (e.g., triphenyl phosphate) have been identified and total about 0.3% of the distillation residue (Vicedo et al., 1985).

Commercial hexane (containing about 30% *n*-hexane) has a slightly disagreeable odour, perceptible at 282 mg/m^3 (80 ppm) (intermittent exposure) or 528 mg/m^3 (150 ppm) (continuous exposure) (Patty & Yant, 1929). An odour threshold of 211 mg/m^3 (60 ppm) for hexane (purity not stated) has also been reported (Laffort & Dravnieks, 1973).

2.3 Conversion factors

1 ppm *n*-hexane in air = 3.52 mg/m^3
1 mg/m^3 = 0.284 ppm *n*-hexane in air

2.4 Analytical methods

n-Hexane may be analysed by gas chromatography with flame ionization detection or mass spectroscopy. A summary of the techniques employed is given in Table 3.

Carbon cloth can be used for diffusive sampling. It has been shown that when it is wrapped in aluminium foil there is no significant loss of *n*-hexane during storage for at least four days (Kasahara & Ikeda, 1987).

A high performance liquid chromatographic method using a silica cartridge has been developed for the analysis of *n*-hexane metabolites (2-hexanone, 2,5-dimethylfuran, γ-valerolactone, 5-hydroxy-2-hexanone, and 2,5-hexanedione) in chicken plasma (Nomeir & Abou-Donia 1985). Metabolites of *n*-hexane have also been analysed by gas chromatography coupled with mass spectroscopy (DiVincenzo et al, 1976).

Table 3. Techniques for the analysis of *n*-hexane

Medium	Separation method	Detection system	Limit of sensitivity	Reference
Air	trap with charcoal; desorb with CS_2; steel column; gas chromatography (FFAP)	flame ionization	validated over the range 877-3679 mg/m^3 at 17 °C, 764 mmHg; probable useful range: 180-5400 mg/m^3	NIOSH (1977b)
Air	trap with charcoal; desorb with CS_2; gas chromatography	flame ionization	measurement range: 3.56-14.5 mg for 5-μl injection	NIOSH (1984)
Air	diffusive sampling; thermal desorption	stain tube (Kitagawa 133 5B)	detection range: 18-500 μg	Gentry & Walsh (1987)
Liquid	glass column; gas chromatography; 5% carbowax (partition) or 0.3% carbowax (adsorption)	flame ionization	not given	Franke et al. (1988)
Liquid	capillary glass column; gas chromatography (OV101)	flame ionization	0.05 μg	Nomeir & Abou-Donia (1985)
Biological samples	glass column; gas chromatography (Porapak Q)	mass spectrometer (multiple ion monitoring m/z 85)	80 ng/g (biological sample)	Tsuruta (1980)

3. SOURCES OF HUMAN AND ENVIRONMENTAL EXPOSURE

3.1 Natural occurrence

n-Hexane is present in natural gas and crude oil (Guthrie 1960).

3.2 Production and uses

3.2.1 Production levels and processes

3.2.1.1 Production figures

It has been estimated that 306 000 tonnes of *n*-hexane was recovered from petroleum and natural gas in 1977 in the USA (Dale & Montgomery, 1983). Babich et al. (1982) cited approximate estimates of 240 000 to 465 000 tonnes (80-155 million gallons) for the annual production of naphtha (of which hexane is the principal component) in the USA in 1978/1979, and the total production in the USA in 1987 was 386 500 tonnes (USITC, 1988).

3.2.1.2 Manufacturing processes

Two-tower distillation of a suitable hydrocarbon feed-stock is used for the manufacture of commercial hexanes. The feedstock may be straight-run gasolines distilled from crude oil or natural gas liquids stripped of natural gas. Hexanes can also be obtained from the remains of catalytic reformates after the removal of aromatics. Very pure *n*-hexane can be produced from hexane mixtures by adsorption on molecular sieves (Dale & Drehman, 1983).

3.2.2 Uses

In most cases, *n*-hexane is used as a mixture with other hexane isomers and various solvents. The following uses of *n*-hexane have been reported (Dale & Drehman, 1983; CCOHS, 1985):

- in food processing, including the extraction of vegetable oil from soybeans, flaxseed, peanuts, safflower seed, corngerm, and cottonseed;
- as a polyolefins solvent and as a cleaning agent;
- as a rubber polymerization solvent;
- as a laboratory chemical;
- in low-temperature thermometers;
- in the manufacture of pharmaceuticals;
- in other products (e.g., adhesives, lacquers).

The consumption of hexane (not specifically *n*-hexane) in the USA and Canada during 1975 for the above purposes was estimated to be 450 000 to 490 000 m^3 (120-130 million gallons) (Dale & Drehman, 1983). The consumption of *n*-hexane in the EEC in 1979 was 10 000 tonnes.

In general, petroleum distillate solvents of a relatively low boiling point contain a relatively high proportion of *n*-hexane (Kasahara et al., 1987). Rubber surface softener samples and approximately one half of the analysed samples of thinner-cleaner used for printing and painting were in this category (Kasahara et al., 1987). Ikeda & Kasahara (1986) found the *n*-hexane content to be 0.4-9% in four samples of gasoline with boiling points in the range 30-160 °C.

4. ENVIRONMENTAL TRANSPORT, DISTRIBUTION, AND TRANSFORMATION

4.1 Transport and distribution between media

There is little information on the transport and mobility of *n*-hexane in the environment. It is very insoluble in water (9.5 mg/litre at 25 °C) (McAuliffe, 1963), and transport occurs predominantly in the vapour phase once it is emitted into the environment. The solubility of *n*-hexane in water is increased by the presence of methanol (Groves, 1988).

Chiou et al. (1988) determined that the sorptive capacity of soil for hexane is 11 mg/g (0.0167 ml/g).

4.2 Biotransformation and photochemical reactivity

Information is only available on the abiotic degradation of *n*-hexane. Atmospheric *n*-hexane is not expected to have a pronounced effect on the physical properties of the atmosphere, to participate in the depletion of the ozone layer, or to alter precipitation patterns (CIIT, 1977). The rate constant for the reaction of hydroxyl (OH) radicals with *n*-hexane was determined (using a smog chamber) to be 6.2 ($\pm$ 0.6) x 10^{-12} cm^3 sec^{-1} at 39 °C (Nolting et al., 1988). Other reported values are 5.63 ($\pm$ 0.09) x 10^{-12} cm^3 sec^{-1} at 26 °C (Atkinson et al., 1982) and 5.68 ($\pm$ 0.04) x 10^{-12} cm^3 sec^{-1} (Behnke et al., 1988). In the latter study, there was additional degradation in the presence of titanium dioxide aerosol. These rate coefficients are in good agreement with the value of Klopffer et al. (1988), who measured a K_{OH} of 6.8 x 10^{-12} cm^3 sec^{-1} in a smog chamber at 27 °C. The half-life of *n*-hexane in the troposphere is estimated to be 2 to 2.4 days, based on degradation by OH radicals alone.

Similar hydrocarbons (*n*-pentane and methyl pentane) undergo photochemical conversion to a "smog" containing peroxyacetylnitrate and ozone, but *n*-hexane is one of the least photochemically reactive hydrocarbons (Katagiri & Ohashi, 1975).

5. ENVIRONMENTAL LEVELS AND HUMAN EXPOSURE

5.1 Environmental levels

5.1.1 Air

Fugitive losses of *n*-hexane may occur in industries in which it is used as a solvent or cleaning agent and in the rubber industry. In 1970, prior to the mandatory use of catalytic converters, *n*-hexane was also estimated to represent 1.2% (by volume) of total emitted hydrocarbons from vehicular exhausts in the USA (equivalent to approximately 170 000 tonnes of hexane) (CIIT, 1977). Lonneman et al. (1974) detected *n*-hexane in air samples collected in the Lincoln Tunnel, New York, over a 0.5-h period. *n*-Hexane has been detected at a level of 0.11 mg/m^3 (0.03 ppm) in the ambient atmosphere of Los Angeles (Nelligan, 1962). Hodgson et al. (1986) reported that the concentrations of *n*-hexane in a single open-office space were 1.97 μg/m^3 (0.56 ppb) and 4 μg/m^3 (1.14 ppb) (with 100% ventilation exhaust on and off, respectively), compared with an outdoor concentration that was below the limit of quantification.

In the Federal Republic of Germany, *n*-hexane belongs to class III of chemical substances, the total emission of which (as the sum of all compounds in this class) must not exceed 150 mg/m^3 at a mass flow of 3 kg/h or more (IRPTC, 1990). In the USSR, the ambient vapour concentration of *n*-hexane is regulated at a maximum of 300 mg/m^3 (IRPTC, 1990).

5.1.2 Water

n-Hexane has been detected in the USA in trace quantities in chlorinated tap water derived from a lake (CEC, 1979).

5.1.3 Food

The Joint FAO/WHO Expert Committee on Food Additives (JECFA) has not set an ADI for *n*-hexane but stresses that the solvent should be used only in accordance with good manufacturing practice to ensure minimal residues in food (WHO, 1971). In the USA, cottonseed products and hop extract, modified for human consumption, may contain no more than 60 mg/kg and 25 mg/kg, respectively (CFR, 1987a). The latter limit also applies to certain food colouring agents (CFR, 1987b). The EEC Directive on Extraction Solvents (June 1988) set maximum residue levels in food of between 1 and 30 mg/kg depending on the particular use (IRPTC, 1990).

5.2 Occupational exposure during manufacture, formulation, or use

In addition to the presence of *n*-hexane in the air during its manufacture, a study has indicated detectable levels in air samples from a variety of industrial uses of products containing *n*-hexane. The relative abundance (percentage of samples in which it was detected) was 15% (printing), 7% (painting), 10% (car repair), and 6% (various other operations) (Veulemans et al., 1987). Levels of hexane exposure in six olive extraction plants in Granada, Spain, were found to vary from 3 to 341 mg per m^3 (0.9-97 ppm) (Medinilla & Espigares, 1989). An Italian worker employed at home manufacturing shoes was found to have a urinary 2,5-hexanedione level of 5.7 mg/litre, which exceeded the ACGIH biological exposure index for hexane of 5 mg/litre (Discalzi et al., 1988). Concentrations of *n*-hexane have also been measured in the air to which petroleum service attendants, transport drivers, and outside operators were exposed. For outside operators, 54 out of 56 samples contained measurable concentrations of *n*-hexane, the mean concentration being 0.473 ± 0.594 mg/m^3. All 49 samples of air for transport drivers contained *n*-hexane (mean concentration, 1.019 ± 1.953 mg/m^3). Service attendants were exposed to a mean concentration of 1.175 ± 0.894 mg/m^3 (detected in 48/49 samples). These values represented 2.5, 2.2, and 1.7% of the total hydrocarbon concentration for the three job categories, respectively (Rappaport et al., 1987). Maximum time-weighted average (8 h) concentrations of hexane at a hexane extraction facility were found to be 92 mg/m^3 (26 ppm) (NIOSH, 1981a). NIOSH (1983) reported hexane concentrations in air samples from six breathing zones at a soybean extraction facility that ranged from 15.5 to 46.5

mg/m^3 (4.4-13.2 ppm). In area spot samples, the concentrations were 46.5-94.7 mg/m^3 (13.2-26.9 ppm).

In one metropolitan sewer in Cincinnati, USA, in 1981, the airspace was found to contain hexane at a concentration greater than the lower explosive limit (1.2% by volume in air). Two sewers contained hexane levels of at least 39 600 mg/m^3 (11 250 ppm) (NIOSH, 1981b).

Some limits for occupational exposure in various countries are shown in Table 4. Some countries (e.g., USA, Belgium, and the United Kingdom) also recommend an exposure limit (TWA) of 360 mg/m^3 for all hexane isomers other than *n*-hexane.

Table 4. Some national occupational air exposure limit values[a]

Country/ organization	Exposure limit description[b]	Value	Effective date[c]
Australia	Threshold limit value (TLV)		
	- Time-weighted average (TWA)	360 mg/m^3	1985(r)
Belgium	Threshold limit value (TLV)		
	- Time-weighted average (TWA)	180 mg/m^3	1989(r)
Canada	Threshold limit value (TLV)		
	- Time-weighted average (TWA)	180 mg/m^3	1989
Finland	Maximum permissible concentration (MPC)		
	- Time-weighted average (TWA)	180 mg/m^3	1989(r)
	- Short-term exposure limit (STEL)	530 mg/m^3	
Germany, Federal Republic of	Maximum acceptable concentration (MAK)		
	- Time-weighted average (TWA)	180 mg/m^3	
	- Short-term exposure limit (STEL)	360 mg/m^3	1989(r)
	- Biological tolerance value (BAT) urine: hexane-2,5-dione plus 4,5-dihydroxy-2-haxanone at end of exposure or end of shift	9 mg/litre	
Germany, Democratic Republic of	Maximum acceptable concentration (MAC)		
	- Time-weighted average (TWA)	100 mg/m^3	
	- Short-term exposure limit (STEL)	400 mg/m^3	1988(r)
Italy	Threshold limit value (TLV)		
	- Time-weighted average (TWA)	360 mg/m^3	1985(r)
Japan	Maximum acceptable concentration (MAC)		
	- Time-weighted average (TWA) (skin absorption must also be considered)	141 mg/m^3	1985

Table 4 (contd).

Country/ organization	Exposure limit description[b]	Value	Effective date[c]
Poland	Maximum permissible concentration (MPC) - ceiling value (CLV)	400 mg/m^3	1986(r)
Romania	Maximum permissible concentration (MPC) - Time-weighted average (TWA) - Ceiling value (CLV)	1200 mg/m^3 1500 mg/m^3	1975(r)
Switzerland	Maximum acceptable concentration (MAK) - Time-weighted averge (TWA)	180 mg/m^3	1987
Sweden	Hygienic limit value (HLV) - Time-weighted average (TWA) - Short-term exposure limit (STEL)	90 mg/m^3 180 mg/m^3	1990(n)
United Kingdom	Guidance limit (under review) - Time-weighted average (TWA) - Short-term exposure limit (STEL) (10 min)	360 mg/m^3 450 mg/m^3	1990(n)
USA (ACGIH)	Threshold limit value (TLV) - Time-weighted average (TWA) - Biological exposure index (BEI) 2,5-hexanedione in urine (end of shift) n-hexane in end-exhaled air (during shift)	176 mg/m^3 5 mg/litre 144 mg/m^3	1990(r)
(OSHA)	Permissible exposure limit (PEL)	180 mg/m^3	1990(r)
Yugoslavia	Maximum permissible concentration (MAC) - Time-weighted average (TWA)	1800 mg/m^3	1971(r)

[a] From: IRPTC (1990).
[b] TWA = a maximum mean exposure limit based generally over the period of a working day (usually 8 or 12 h)
STEL = a maximum concentration of exposure for a specified time duration (generally 15 or 30 min).
[c] When no effective date appears in the IRPTC legal file, the year of the reference from which the data are taken is shown, indicated by (r)
n = notified direct by country.

6. KINETICS AND METABOLISM

6.1 Experimental animals

6.1.1 Absorption, distribution, metabolism, and excretion

Radiolabelled ^{14}C-*n*-hexane was absorbed by F-344 rats following inhalation of concentrations of 1760, 3520, 10 560, and 35 200 mg/m^3 (500, 1000, 3000, and 10 000 ppm) for 6 h daily for 3 days (Bus et al., 1982). The proportion of ^{14}C-*n*-hexane recovered in expired air was dose dependent and increased from 12% at 1760 mg/m^3 (500 ppm) to 62% at 35 200 mg/m^3 (10 000 ppm). There was a corresponding decrease in the proportion recovered in urine (from 35% at 1760 mg/m^3 (500 ppm) to 18% at 35 200 mg/m^3 (10 000 ppm), in faeces (from 4.9% at 1760 mg/m^3 (500 ppm) to 0.7% at 35 200 mg/m^3 (10 000 ppm), and in the carcass (from 10% at 1760 mg/m^3 (500 ppm) to 1.5% at 35 200 mg/m^3 (10 000 ppm). The levels of ^{14}C-*n*-hexane in expired air decreased biphasically, with half-lives of 1 and 4.5 h. A biphasic elimination profile was reported for labelled carbon dioxide in exhaled air, the initial half-life being 4.5-7.5 h and 85-96% of the exhaled labelled carbon dioxide being eliminated within 24 h after exposure. Urinary excretion of metabolites also occurred in two phases, most being excreted in the initial phase with a half-life of 7-8 h. The greater part of the radioactivity absorbed during inhalation of *n*-hexane was excreted within 24 h. The rate of metabolism was non-linear above 1056 mg/m^3 (300 ppm) but not below this concentration: it rose from 47 μmol/h per kg body weight at 1056 mg/m^3 (300 ppm) to 245 μmol/h per kg body weight at 10 560 mg/m^3 (3000 ppm). The amount of *n*-hexane in the rat increased in a dose-dependent manner to a limiting value of 9.6 relative to the atmospheric concentration (Filser et al., 1987).

The rate of uptake following inhalation of hexane in male F-344/N rats was found to be 5-7 nmol/kg per min (Dahl et al., 1988). Absorption and distribution into tissues and organs (including blood) was rapid following inhalation exposure of F-344 rats to *n*-hexane (Baker & Rickert, 1981; Howd et al., 1982). Exposure to concentrations between 3520 mg/m^3 and 35 200 mg/m^3 (1000 ppm and 10 000 ppm) resulted in plateau levels of *n*-hexane being reached within 30 min in blood and within 2 h in the other tissues examined (liver, kidney, lungs, testis, brain, and sciatic nerve) (Baker & Rickert, 1981). Acute inhalation exposure to 302 720 mg/m^3 (86 000 ppm) resulted in saturated blood levels within 10 min (Raje et al., 1984).

Dermal absorption of *n*-hexane by guinea-pigs is poor (Jakobson et al., 1982). Tsuruta (1982) measured the penetration of *n*-hexane through excised rat skin and came to a similar conclusion. However, skin absorption of *n*-hexane may be enhanced by other solvents in the mixture. The highest tissue concentrations of *n*-hexane were found in peripheral nerves (sciatic) (Baker & Rickert, 1981; Bus et al., 1981). Steady-state concentrations in blood, sciatic nerve, liver, and lung were directly proportional to the exposure level, but there was some evidence of saturation in the kidney, brain, and testis.

In female albino rats exposed to a hexane level of 17 000 mg/m^3 (50 000 ppm) for up to 10 h, the hexane concentration in the liver increased with time and steady-state levels were not achieved (Böhlen et al., 1973). However, kidney, adrenal, blood, brain, and spleen levels of hexane reached a steady state after approximately 5 h of exposure. The high level of hexane exposure resulted in lipid accumulation in the liver, and, as hexane is highly lipid soluble, this could account for the non-saturability of liver for hexane.

n-Hexane has been detected in the fat, muscle, and bone (sternum) of F-344 rats exposed to an *n*-hexane level of 21 123 mg/m^3 (6800 ppm) for 4 h and in rat fetuses following inhalation exposure of pregnant females (Bus et al., 1979). The concentration in total fetal tissue was similar to that in maternal blood (Babanov & Babanov, 1981).

Elimination of *n*-hexane from rat blood and brain was found to be rapid and multiphasic, with initial half-lives of 2-4 and 7 min and a subsequent half-life of 1-2 h (Bus et al., 1979; White et al., 1979; Baker & Rickert, 1981; Howd et al., 1982). In the rat, elimination from other adult tissues, including sciatic nerve and liver, and from fetal tissue was also rapid but was slower from the kidneys (half-life, 6 h). In the guinea-pig, biphasic elimination from blood (half-lives of 0.5 h and 4 h) has been reported (Couri et al., 1978).

n-Hexane is oxidized to 1-, 2-, or 3-hexanol. 2-Hexanol may be further metabolized to 2-hexanone (methyl-*n*-butyl ketone). 2,5-Hexanediol, 5-hydroxy-2-hexanone, 2,5-hexanedione, γ-valerolactone, 2,5-dimethylfuran, 2,5-dimethyl-2,3-dihydrofuran, 2,5-dimethyltetrahydrofuran, and carbon dioxide have been identified following exposure to *n*-hexane or 2-hexanone. However, furan derivatives and γ-valerolactone are questionable metabolites of *n*-hexane because they may be artefacts (DiVincenzo et al., 1976; Perbellini et al., 1982a; Fedtke & Bolt, 1986b). 2,5-Dimethyl-2,3-dihydrofuran and small amounts of labelled 2-aminohexanoic acid (norleucine), another unidentified amino acid, and urea have been detected following oral dosing of rats with $1-^{14}C-2$-hexanone. Pentanone (isomeric form not specified) has been detected in rat fetuses from dams exposed to 2-hexanone vapour (DiVincenzo et al., 1977; Peters et al., 1981). Radiolabelled 2,5-hexanedione is metabolized to carbon dioxide in the rat (Angelo & Bischoff, 1982). Proposed metabolic pathways for *n*-hexane in mammals are shown in Fig. 1.

2-Hexanol was the major urinary metabolite excreted by rats during *n*-hexane inhalation exposure for up to 24 h (Perbellini et al., 1982a; Iwata et al., 1983b). After exposure, the main urinary metabolites were 2,5-hexanedione, 2,5-dimethylfuran, and γ-valerolactone (Baker & Rickert, 1981; Perbellini et al., 1982a; Iwata et al., 1983b). All the γ-valerolactone and a significant proportion of the other metabolites were conjugated; glucuronides of 2-hexanol and 2,5-dimethylfuran were identified. Only small amounts of 2-hexanone, 5-hydroxy-2-hexanone, and 3-hexanol were present. 1-Hexanol, mainly as the glucuronide, has been detected following intraperitoneal injection of *n*-hexane (Dolara et al., 1978). With prolonged exposure to 1760 mg/m³ (500 ppm) (3 h/day, for 33 weeks), 80-90% of all urinary metabolites were conjugated, the predominant metabolites being 2-hexanol and 2,5-hexanedione (Iwata et al., 1984). In urine collected from rats during and up to 24 h after exposure to 3520 mg

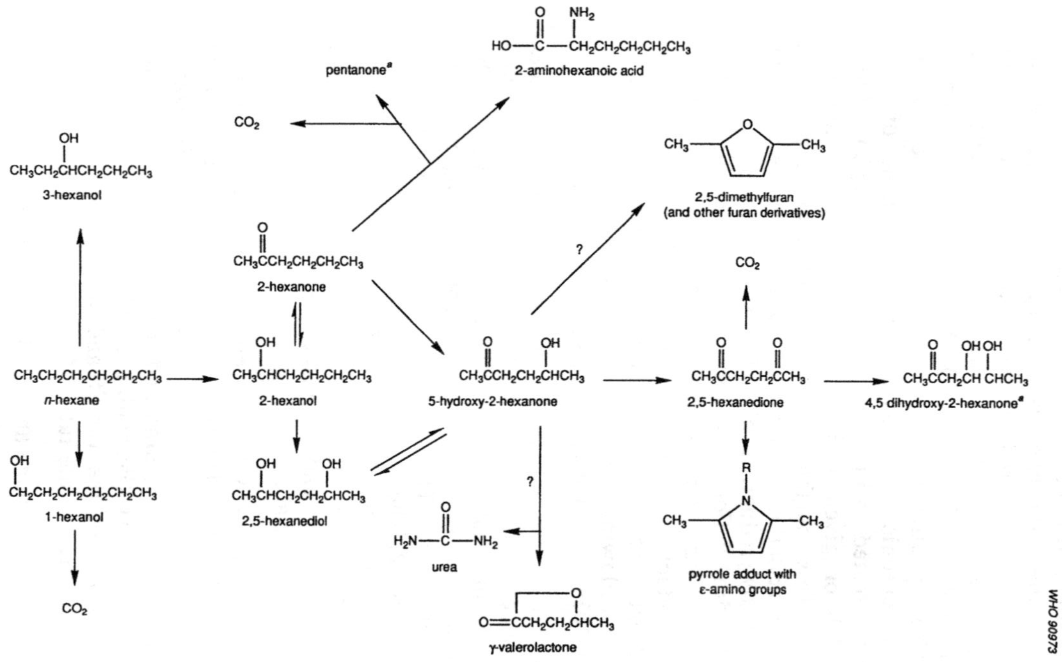

Fig. 1. Proposed metabolic pathways of n-hexane in animals

[a] Isometric form not specified in original report.

? Some investigators have questioned the validity of these pathways.

[b] Possibly via 5-hydroxy-2-hexanone

per m³ (1000 ppm), the predominant urinary metabolites were 2-hexanol and 2,5-hexanedione, of which 99 and 90%, respectively, were found (following acid hydrolysis) to be conjugated. In addition, all the 1-hexanol and 3-hexanol and 30% of the 2-hexanol were conjugated. The hexanol conjugates were considered to be glucuronides and sulfate esters, but the identity of the other conjugates was unclear (Fedtke & Bolt, 1986b). Subsequently, Fedtke & Bolt (1987a) identified 4,5-dihydroxy-2-hexanone as an additional glucuronic acid conjugate in the urine of male Wistar rats treated with *n*-hexane at 7040 mg/m³ (2000 ppm) for 8 h or given a single ip dose of 2,5-hexanedione (200 mg/kg). This metabolite was considered to be produced either by hydroxylation of 5-hydroxy-2-hexanone (which may be produced by reduction of 2,5-hexanedione) or alternatively by hydroxylation and subsequent reduction of 2,5-hexanedione. Thus, 4,5-dihydroxy-2-hexanone may be a detoxified product of 2,5-hexanedione. This metabolite was the second most abundant metabolite in the urine of male Wistar rats following inhalation of *n*-hexane (176-10 820 mg/m³, 50-3074 ppm) for 8 h (Fedtke & Bolt, 1987b).

In studies on the rabbit and monkey *(Macaca mulatta),* the urinary excretion of *n*-hexane metabolites was found to differ from that of rats (Perbellini et al., 1982b). 2-Hexanol was the main urinary metabolite during and after inhalation exposure. The other metabolites present were 3-hexanol and 2,5-hexanedione; γ-valerolactone and 2,5-dimethylfuran were not detected. Following intraperitoneal injection of *n*-hexane in guinea-pigs, 2-hexanol, mainly as the glucuronide, and *n*-hexane itself were identified in the urine (Couri et al., 1978).

Elimination half-lives in rat urine for individual metabolites following inhalation of *n*-hexane have been determined for 2-hexanone (4 h), 3-hexanol and 2,5-hexanedione (7 h), 2,5-dimethylfuran and γ-valerolactone (11-14 h), and 2-hexanol (18 h) (Perbellini et al., 1982a). The half-life for 2-hexanol in the rabbit and monkey was found to be shorter (8 h) than in the rat.

5-Hydroxy-2-hexanone and 2,5-hexanedione were detected in guinea-pig serum after intraperitoneal administration of *n*-hexane (DiVincenzo et al., 1976). Following administration of 2-hexanol, a major urinary metabolite of *n*-hexane in some species, two additional compounds, 2-hexanone and 2,5-hexanediol, were found. A similar metabolic profile was found following the administration of 2-hexanone, with 5-hydroxy-2-hexanone, 2,5-hexanedione, and 2-hexanol being identified as metabolites. 2,5-Hexanedione, which is considered to be the active neurotoxic agent, can thus be formed from *n*-hexane, 2-hexanol, or 2-hexanone.

6.1.2 Kinetics of 2,5-hexanedione

A marked increase in blood levels of 2,5-hexanedione on inhalation exposure to *n*-hexane at 3168 or 17 600 mg/m³ (900 or 5000 ppm) for 6-24 h has been observed in separate studies (Perbellini et al., 1982a; Kulig, 1983; Kulig et al., 1984). No evidence of 2,5-hexanedione accumulation in blood was found in Wistar rats after repeated exposures to *n*-hexane at 3168 mg/m³ (900 ppm), 8 h/day, for 9 days (Kulig, 1983). 2,5-Hexanedione was completely eliminated, within 6.25 h of the end of exposure, from the blood of Wistar rats exposed to an *n*-hexane level of 3168 mg/m³ (900 ppm) 8 h/day, for 72 weeks (De Groot & Kepner, 1984). There was no significant difference in 2,5-hexanedione blood levels in Fischer 344 rats exposed for 1 or 5 days to 3520 mg/m³ (1000 ppm) for 6 h/day (Bus et al., 1981). In contrast, there were significantly increased 2,5-hexanedione concentrations in the blood of Fischer-344 rats after 3 exposures to 14 080 mg/m³ (4000 ppm) for 8 h/day compared with a single 8-h exposure (Howd et al., 1982).

The elimination half-life for 2,5-hexanedione from blood has been reported to vary between different strains of rat. Values for Sprague-Dawley and Fischer-344 rats were 2.3 h and 3.9-6 h, respectively, and an initial half-life of 1 h has been reported for Wistar rats (Bus et al., 1979; Angelo & Bischoff, 1982; Howd et al., 1982; Kulig, 1983). It has been suggested that differences in the rates of elimination of 2,5-hexanedione from the blood may explain the reported greater susceptibility to *n*-hexane-induced neurotoxicity of Fischer-344 rats compared with Wistar rats (Kulig, 1983; Kulig et al., 1984).

In a study by Ladefoged & Perbellini (1986), 2,5-hexanedione (50 mg/kg) was administered to five male rabbits by intravenous injection. The pharmacokinetic data fitted a two-compartment model in which the half-life was 42 (± 11) min (body clearance was 0.0117 (± 0.0026) ml/min per kg).

Blood concentrations of 2,5-hexanedione have been estimated following continuous exposure of rats to *n*-hexane (Kulig, 1983; Kulig et al., 1984). Marked reductions in blood 2,5-hexanedione levels were reported following exposure to 3168 mg/m^3 (900 ppm) for 3 days compared with one day. There were no further decreases after 9 or 20 days of exposure. Smaller reductions were observed in short-term studies after 8 or 12 weeks of exposure to 3168 mg/m^3 (900 ppm) for either 8 or 24 h/day, 5 days per week, compared with the blood levels of 2,5-hexanedione recorded after 4 weeks of exposure to 3168 mg/m^3 (900 ppm). No effects were reported in similar short-term studies at 1056 mg/m^3 (300 ppm) (Kulig, 1983). This may be due to the enhancement of glucuronidation (a major elimination pathway) by hexane, a phenomenon noted in both *in vitro* and *in vivo* studies in the guinea-pig (Notten & Henderson, 1975a,b). Similar levels of 2,5-hexanedione in blood were found in weanling and young adult rats following one week of continuous exposure to 3520 mg/m^3 (1000 ppm) (Pryor et al., 1982).

2,5-Hexanedione was detected in the blood, sciatic nerve, brain, kidneys, liver, and lungs, but not in the testes, following exposure of Fischer-344 rats to levels of *n*-hexane between 1760 and 35 200 mg/m^3 (500 to 10 000 ppm) for 6 h (Baker & Rickert, 1981). The relationship between peak tissue concentrations of 2,5-hexanedione and *n*-hexane exposure levels was complex. In the kidneys, sciatic nerve, and brain, the highest concentrations were obtained after exposure to 3520 mg/m^3 (1000 ppm). In a further study, lower tissue levels and greater elimination of 2,5-hexanedione were found in mice than in rats after a single exposure to 3520 mg/m^3 (1000 ppm) for 6 h (Baker et al., 1980).

The elimination of 2,5-hexanedione from the rat liver, kidney, brain, and sciatic nerve was determined after exposure to 3520 mg/m^3 (1000 ppm) 6 h/day, for 1 or 5 days (Bus et al., 1981). 2,5-Hexanedione was selectively retained in sciatic nerve but not in the brain. However, comparable rates of elimination of 2,5-hexanedione from the brain, sciatic nerve, and blood were reported in Sprague-Dawley rats given a single oral dose of 2,5-hexanedione (Iwasaki & Tsuruta, 1984). Terminal half-lives of 32-33 days were reported in a review of some earlier studies (O'Donoghue, 1985).

2,5-Hexanedione has also been detected in fetal tissue, at a level similar to that in maternal blood, following exposure of F-344 rats to *n*-hexane (Bus et al., 1979). A fetal half-life of 3 h was calculated.

Less than 10% of 2,5-hexanedione in blood is bound to plasma components (Angelo & Bischoff, 1982). A study on hens dosed orally with 2,5-hexanedione showed that it can form a pyrrole adduct with serum protein (DeCaprio et al., 1982).

6.1.3 In vitro studies

n-Hexane penetrates excised rat skin slowly (Tsuruta, 1977, 1982).

In rat liver and lung preparations, *n*-hexane has been shown to be hydroxylated to 1-, 2-, and 3-hexanol (Frommer et al., 1974; Walseth et al., 1982; Toftgard et al., 1984). 2-Hexanol was found to be the predominant metabolite, and 2,5-hexanedione was also formed in studies with rat liver microsomes (Frommer et al., 1974; Walseth et al., 1982). More than one form of cytochrome P-450 is involved in *n*-hexane oxidation (Frommer et al., 1974). In the rat lung the formation of 2- and 3-hexanol is catalysed by a different microsomal cytochrome P-450 isoenzyme (cytochrome P-450-PB-B) from that responsible for the formation of 1-hexanol (Toftgard et al., 1984). Toftgard et al. (1984, 1986) found that rat liver microsomes, but not lung microsomes, contained a cytochrome P-450 isoenzyme that converted 2-hexanol to 2,5-hexanediol, and that the oxidation of hexanols and 2,5-hexanediol by alcohol dehydrogenase was restricted to the liver. These results suggest that, during inhalation of *n*-hexane, the metabolite 2,5-hexanedione is likely to be formed in the liver but not in the lung.

Preparations of purified rabbit liver cytochrome P-450 hydroxylate *n*-hexane, and mouse liver microsomes hydroxylate hexane (Ichihara et al., 1969; Nilsen et al., 1981). Studies using liver fractions from guinea-pigs demonstrated that *n*-hexane can be metabolized to 2-hexanol, 2-hexanone, and 2,5-hexanedione (Couri et al., 1978). 2-Hexanone was reduced to 2-hexanol by the cytosolic fraction and oxidized to 2,5-hexanedione by the microsomal fraction.

In mouse nerve and muscle tissue cultures, *n*-hexane was metabolized to 2-hexanediol and 2,5-hexanedione, and 5-hydroxy-2-hexanone was detected following incubation with 2-hexanol or 2-hexanone (Veronesi et al., 1978, 1980; Spencer et al., 1980).

2,5-Hexanedione has been found to react with primary amino groups in proteins, such as the ε-amino group of lysine, to yield 2,5-dimethylpyrrole adducts (DeCaprio et al., 1982; Graham et al., 1982a,b). Pyrrole formation is an obligatory step in the pathogenesis of neuropathy caused by *n*-hexane (Sayre et al., 1986). 2,5-Hexanedione appears to be the active neurotoxic metabolite of *n*-hexane.

6.1.4 Effects of other chemicals on n-hexane metabolism

Urinary excretion of *n*-hexane metabolites by rats has been shown to be increased following pre-treatment with phenobarbital, an inducer of the microsomal oxidation of foreign compounds by cytochrome P-450 isoenzymes (Perbellini et al., 1979, 1982a).

In *in vitro* studies, pre-treatment of rats with phenobarbital increased the extent of liver microsomal oxidation of *n*-hexane to 2- and 3-hexanol, and pre-treatment with another inducer, 3,4-benzo[*a*]pyrene, enhanced 3-hexanol formation (Frommer et al., 1974; Näslund & Halpert, 1984). However, phenobarbital pre-treatment of rats had no effect on *n*-hexane metabolism by lung microsomes (Näslund & Halpert, 1984). Phenobarbital pre-treatment of guinea-pigs increased the metabolism of *n*-hexane to 2-hexanol and 2,5-hexanedione by hepatic post-mitochondrial supernatant, and increased the metabolism of 2-hexanone to 2,5-hexanedione by the hepatic microsomal fraction (Couri et al., 1978).

Intraperitoneal injection of phthalate esters to rats affects the metabolism of *n*-hexane *in vitro*, presumably by induction of cytochrome P-450 (Walseth et al., 1982). Treatment with dimethylphthalate or dibutylphthalate increased significantly the rate of formation of 2- and 3-hexanol by liver microsomes but decreased slightly their formation by lung microsomes. A large increase in 2,5-hexanedione formation by both types of microsomes was noted following exposure to di(2-ethylhexyl)phthalate. Similar results have been reported with inhalation exposures to dibutylphthalate (Walseth & Nilsen, 1984). Male Sprague-Dawley rats were exposed continuously for 5 days to atmospheric dibutylphthalate concentrations of 5.7, 28.5, and 79.7 mg/m³ (0.5, 2.5, and 7 ppm), and liver and lung microsomal fractions were prepared. The *in vitro* formation of *n*-hexane metabolites was assayed by incubating 50 ml of 8% (v/v) *n*-hexane in sodium phosphate buffer with 1 mg lung or liver microsomal protein for 10 min. The formation of 1-, 2-, and 3-hexanol was markedly increased with liver microsomes but not with lung microsomes. At the intermediate and high exposure concentrations of 28.5 and 79.7 mg/m³ (2.5 and 7 ppm), there was a decrease in *in vitro* *n*-hexane metabolism particularly in lung microsomes.

The formation of 1-, 2-, and 3-hexanol from *n*-hexane was significantly increased with kidney and liver microsomes obtained from rats previously exposed to isopropanol (Zahlsen et al., 1985). Enhanced formation of 2- and 3-hexanol (greater in male than in female rats), but not of 1-hexanol, occurred when *n*-hexane was incubated with liver microsomes from rats previously exposed to xylene (mixed isomers) (Toftgard et al., 1983).

Treatment of rats with chloramphenicol (100 mg/kg intraperitoneal or intravenous) inhibited 2- and 3-hexanol formation *in vitro* by lung and liver microsomes derived from these animals (Näslund & Halpert, 1984).

Toluene has been shown to be a non-competitive inhibitor of *n*-hexane metabolism in *in vitro* studies with rat liver preparations (Perbellini et al., 1982b). Exposure of rats to mixtures of *n*-hexane and toluene resulted in reduced urinary excretion of *n*-hexane metabolites (Perbellini et al., 1982b; Iwata et al., 1983b, 1984). However, no effect on blood *n*-hexane levels was reported when rats were given an intraperitoneal *n*-hexane injection of 0.91 g/kg with or without 1.18 g toluene/kg (Suzuki et al., 1974). In a study on the kinetics of 2,5-hexanedione (section 6.1.2), Ladefoged & Perbellini (1986) dosed six male rabbits intravenously with 50 mg 2,5-hexanedione/kg with or without acetone (150 mg/kg). A significant reduction of 2,5-hexanedione clearance was caused by the acetone co-treatment.

Blood levels of 2,5-hexanedione were reduced after a single 6-h co-exposure to *n*-hexane (3520 mg/m^3, 1000 ppm) and methyl ethyl ketone (2950 mg/m^3, 1000 ppm), but not in animals pre-treated orally with methyl ethyl ketone. However, pre-treatment resulted in increases in liver cytochrome P-450 levels and in reactions mediated by mixed-function oxidase (Robertson et al., 1982; Robertson et al., 1989). Lower levels of 2,5-hexanedione have been observed in the rat sciatic nerve after exposure to mixtures of *n*-hexane and methyl ethyl ketone, but full data were not presented (White & Bus, 1980).

In studies by Ralston et al. (1985), the blood and tissue clearance of 2,5-hexanedione was measured after single or repeated oral administration of 2,5-hexanedione or of a mixture of equimolar doses of 2,5-hexanedione and methyl ethyl ketone. There was reduced blood elimination of 2,5-hexanedione after administration of the mixture only. The increased blood bioavailability correlated with neurophysiological findings in co-exposed animals. The results suggest that methyl ethyl ketone increases the persistence of 2,5-hexanedione in the blood. Levels of radiolabelled 2,5-hexanedione in neurofilament-enriched preparations from the sciatic nerve and spinal cord were generally unaffected by concurrent exposure to methyl ethyl ketone during the first two weeks of treatment, and a trend towards decreased tissue levels was evident after 3 weeks.

Reduced urinary excretion of *n*-hexane metabolites has been reported in rats following exposure to mixtures of *n*-hexane and methyl ethyl ketone (Perbellini et al., 1982b; Iwata et al., 1983b, 1984). The effect appeared to be transitory and no significant effects remained after 33 weeks of co-exposure. In contrast, increased urinary excretion of 2,5-hexanedione was observed in guinea-pigs exposed to mixtures of methyl ethyl ketone and 2-hexanone (Couri et al., 1978).

6.2 Human beings

The disposition and metabolism of *n*-hexane have been studied in human beings following exposure by inhalation and skin contact. Most studies were conducted on workers occupationally exposed to commercial hexane and thus exposed to varying levels of cyclohexane, 2-methylpentane, and 3-methylpentane, as well as *n*-hexane; significant levels of methyl ethyl ketone and toluene have also been recorded. Three experimental studies on human volunteers presumably used pure *n*-hexane (Nomiyama & Nomiyama, 1974a,b; Ralston et al., 1985; Filser et al., 1987). *n*-Hexane is absorbed following inhalation (Nomiyama & Nomiyama, 1974a,b; Brugnone et al., 1978, 1980; Veulemans et al., 1982; Mutti et al., 1984; Perbellini et al., 1985a). Steady-state pulmonary retention (calculated by measuring the percentage of hexane in inhaled and expired air) was in the region of 15-30%, and there was no evidence of saturation at concentrations of up to 704 mg/m^3 (200 ppm). Pulmonary retention was greater in more obese individuals, and, although the alveolar uptake rate decreased during physical exercise, the total uptake of *n*-hexane increased slightly as a result of the higher lung ventilation rate. A net lung uptake of 112 mg in 8 h was reported in workers exposed to an *n*-hexane level of 180 mg/m^3 (51 ppm) (Perbellini et al., 1985a). Alveolar air concentrations of *n*-hexane correlated with blood concentrations in industrial workers exposed to commercial hexane (Brugnone et al., 1984).

Some *n*-hexane is exhaled following cessation of exposure (Nomiyama & Nomiyama, 1974b), and it has been suggested that this amounts to about 10% of the net amount absorbed (Mutti et al., 1984). Elimination was rapid and biphasic, with half-lives of 0.2 and 1.7 h. Steady-state levels of *n*-hexane in blood were linearly dose dependent following inhalation of up to 704 mg/m^3 (200 ppm) (Veulemans et al., 1982). Near-plateau levels were obtained within 15 min, both in resting volunteers and in those undergoing physical exercise. Following the end of exposure, elimination of *n*-hexane from blood was rapid and biphasic; two half-lives were obtained, one of approximately 0.2 h and the other of 1.5-2 h.

The percutaneous absorption of *n*-hexane in humans has not been well studied, although this route of exposure has been implicated in case reports of peripheral neuropathy (Nomiyama et al., 1973; Takahashi et al., 1977). In a limited study, no hexane was detected in the blood or exhaled air of a volunteer who immersed one hand in *n*-hexane for 1 min (Nomiyama & Nomiyama, 1975).

Filser et al. (1987) measured an *n*-hexane metabolic clearance of 2.2 litres/min at a concentration of approximately 3.52 mg/m^3 (1 ppm) (steady-state concentration), and *n*-hexane accumulated to a factor of 2.3. At low concentrations, the clearance of *n*-hexane was not limited by saturation of metabolism but rather by the rate of transport by the blood to the metabolic system. *n*-Hexane tissue/gas partition coefficients were determined *in vitro* using tissue samples obtained from autopsy cases (Perbellini et al., 1985b). Values for heart, muscle, brain, kidney, and liver ranged from 2.8 to 5.2, whereas the fat/air partition coefficient was 104. The blood/air partition coefficient was 0.8. A half-life of 64 h for *n*-hexane in fat has been calculated from a mathematical model of hexane distribution (Perbellini et al., 1986).

The metabolism of *n*-hexane in humans is qualitatively similar to that in the rat. 2,5-Hexanedione, 2,5-dimethylfuran, γ-valerolactone, and small amounts of 2-hexanol have been identified in urine samples from workers exposed to *n*-hexane (Perbellini & Brugnone, 1980; Perbellini et al., 1981a,b,c,d; Iwata et al., 1983b; Mutti et al., 1984). All these compounds were present as conjugates, together with some free 2,5-hexanedione and 2,5-dimethylfuran (Perbellini & Brugnone, 1980; Perbellini et al., 1981c). The total amounts of these compounds in urine accounted for only 15% of the estimated uptake of *n*-hexane (Mutti et al., 1984). Fedtke & Bolt (1987b) have also identified 4,5-dihydroxy-2-hexanone as a major metabolite in the urine of a male volunteer exposed to *n*-hexane at a level of 764 mg/m^3 (217 ppm) for 4 h. These authors pointed out that the acid hydrolysis commonly used in urine analysis may lead to the actual production of 2,5-hexanedione and 2,5-dimethylfuran from 4,5-dihydroxy-2-hexanone glucuronide. This finding needs to be taken into account for the measurement of urinary 2,5-hexanedione in biological monitoring.

Radiolabelled carbon dioxide has been found in the exhaled air of volunteers after an oral dose of $1\text{-}^{14}C\text{-}2\text{-}$hexanone (DiVincenzo et al., 1978). As 2-hexanone is a metabolite of *n*-hexane, the latter may also be converted to carbon dioxide and exhaled.

The end-of-shift urine concentration of *n*-hexane correlates strongly with the time-weighted average (TWA) *n*-hexane air concentration. Imbriani et al. (1984a,b) reported that 2 h after exposure had ended, urinary concentrations of *n*-hexane were reduced to trace levels. 2,5-Hexanedione was detected in the urine following exposure to a time-weighted average concentration of *n*-hexane in air of more than 53 mg/m^3 (15 ppm) (Iwata et al., 1983b). The end-of-shift urine concentration of 2,5-hexanedione showed a positive correlation with both the *n*-hexane time-weighted average concentration and end-of-shift blood levels of *n*-hexane (Perbellini et al., 1981b, 1985a; Iwata et al., 1983b; Mutti et al., 1984; Ahonen & Schimberg, 1988). A mean half-life of 13 to 14 h for urinary excretion of 2,5-hexanedione has been reported (Mutti et al., 1980; Perbellini et al., 1985a). Urinary excretion of 2,5-hexanedione was greatest 3-5 h after a shift. The end-of-shift level was similar to that of the next morning and was highest at the end of the working week. This finding, and the high partition coefficient and calculated long half-life of *n*-hexane in fat, led to the conclusion that *n*-hexane may accumulate in the human body. The level of urinary 2,5-hexanedione excretion was also positively correlated with the airborne concentration of methyl ethyl ketone. However, it is likely that the individuals with the highest exposure to methyl ethyl ketone also had the highest *n*-hexane exposure, so that the increased urinary 2,5-hexanedione may not be the result of an effect of methyl ethyl ketone on *n*-hexane metabolism. De Rosa et al. (1988) examined 20 workers exposed to *n*-hexane and other solvents during glueing operations in shoe factories. The end-of-shift concentrations of 2,5-hexanedione in the urine correlated (r = 0.87) with the 8-h time-weighted average *n*-hexane exposure (measured as four sequential 2-h samples). A biological exposure index of 4.21 mg/litre was obtained for urine collection on a Thursday, but it was indicated that the index may vary depending on the day of analysis. Ahonen & Schimberg

(1988) estimated a reference value for 2,5-hexanedione of 10 μmol/litre (approximately 0.7 mmol/mol creatinine), corresponding to an 8-h time-weighted average n-hexane concentration of 176 mg/m³ (50 ppm) on the sampling day. This value of 2,5-hexanedione represents the difference between the post-shift and pre-shift samples.

Governa et al. (1987) detected 2,5-hexanedione and γ-valerolactone in the urine of all of 40 shoe factory workers exposed to n-hexane. 2,5-Hexanedione was the major metabolite in 39 of the 40 cases. 2-Hexanol was found in 11 cases and in one case a low level of 2-methyl-2-pentanol was detected. The level of 2,5-hexanedione and γ-valerolactone gave a statistically significant correlation with concomitant electroneuromyographic changes characteristic of neuropathy and the former metabolite was considered a suitable predictive measurement.

Ghittori et al. (1987) found that the urinary concentration (C_u) of n-hexane in exposed workers could be expressed by the following equation:

$$C_u = (0.05 \times C_a) + 3.97$$

where C_a is the time-weighted average environmental air concentration. The 4-h exposure urinary concentration value in workers exposed to a time-weighted average concentration of 180 mg/m³ was 13 μg/litre, whereas the ACGIH biological equivalent exposure limit is 9 μg/litre.

2,5-Hexanedione has also be detected in the urine (0.45 ($\pm$ 0.20) mg/litre) of people apparently not exposed to n-hexane. It was speculated that n-hexane may be produced in the body via lipid peroxidation (Fedtke & Bolt, 1986a).

7. EFFECTS ON ORGANISMS IN THE ENVIRONMENT

There is a lack of information on the effects of *n*-hexane on organisms in the environment. Sax (1984) reported that > 1000 mg/litre is required to kill 50% of exposed "aquatic organisms", but gave no details of species or exposure. Bringmann & Kühn (1982) gave an LC_{50} of > 1000 mg/litre for the waterflea *Daphnia magna*. This was a static test with no measurement of actual exposure concentration. Bobra et al. (1983) reported an LC_{50} for *Daphnia magna* of 3.88 mg/litre, but the test was conducted over 48 h in a vessel closed with an airtight cap. However, it is unlikely that organisms in the natural environment would ever be exposed to *n*-hexane continuously over this period, because the highly volatile *n*-hexane with its low water solubility would rapidly be lost from water. Juhnke & Ludemann (1978) reported LC_{50} values for golden orfe *(Leuciscus melanotus)* of 150-4480 mg/litre. It appears that this was a static test without measurement of actual exposure; the test was reported to have lasted 48 h with "continuous aeration", and results, therefore, should be treated with caution. Stratton & Smith (1988) demonstrated a 50% reduction in the growth of a culture of the green alga *Chlorella pyrenoidosa* in the presence of hexane at 2.66% (v/v) (confidence limits 1.97-3.35%). Hexane had a knock-down effect on the house fly *(Musca domestica L.)* of 7, 20, 47, and 87% 2 h after a topical application of 0.25, 0.5, 1.9, and 2 µl/insect, respectively (Singh & Jain, 1987). The respective mortality rates after 5 h were 0, 20, 60, and 80% and at 24 h were 0, 13, 53, and 87%.

8. EFFECTS ON EXPERIMENTAL ANIMALS AND *IN VITRO* TEST SYSTEMS

8.1 Single exposures

8.1.1 Inhalation exposure

A 1-h LC_{50} value of 271 040 mg/m^3 (77 000 ppm) has been reported for adult Fischer male rats (Pryor et al., 1982). A 4-h LC_{50} value for hexane of 260 480 mg/m^3 (74 000 ppm) was reported in Long-Evans male rats (Hine & Zuidema, 1970), but it was later estimated that the concentration of *n*-hexane in the test material was probably only about 45% (Delbrück & Kluge, 1982). In mice (strain unspecified) exposed to pure *n*-hexane for 2 h, 100 mg per litre was reported to be the minimum lethal concentration (Lazarev, 1929). Anaesthesia occurred in Swiss mice within 1 min of exposure to an *n*-hexane (99% pure) concentration of 225 280 mg/m^3 (64 000 ppm) and respiratory arrest occurred within 4.5 min (Swann et al., 1974). In mice (strain unspecified) exposed to hexane, deaths occurred at concentrations above 133 760 mg/m^3 (38 000 ppm), normally preceded by loss of postural reflexes. The toxicity of inhaled hexane, as measured by its lethality, increased with elevation of temperature from 20 °C to 35 °C (Babanov et al., 1988).

Male Fischer rats exposed by inhalation to *n*-hexane showed myoclonic seizures and ataxia at concentrations above 168 960 mg/m^3 (48 000 ppm) (Pryor et al., 1982). Sprague-Dawley rats showed ataxia and decreased motor activity after 25-30 min exposure to concentrations between 302 720 and 316 800 mg/m^3 (86 000 and 90 000 ppm) (Honma, 1983). Sedation, hypothermia, and ptosis followed exposure of male Sprague-Dawley rats to 7040, 14 080, and 28 160 mg *n*-hexane/m^3 (2000, 4000, and 8000 ppm) for 8 h (Raje et al., 1984). No acute behavioural effects were noted in rats exposed to 84 480 mg/m^3 (24 000 ppm) for 10 min (Pryor et al., 1982). In Swiss mice, light anaesthesia followed exposure to 56 320 mg/m^3 (16 000 ppm) for 5 min, and deep anaesthesia, with periods of apnoea, occurred during exposure to 112 640 mg/m^3 (32 000 ppm) for the same length of time (Swann et al., 1974).

Histopathological effects on the lung (lamellar inclusions in type II pneumocytes) were observed in Wistar rats exposed to an *n*-hexane (96-99% pure) level of 35 200 mg/m³ (10 000 ppm) for 4 or 8 h or to 24 640 mg/m³ (700 ppm) for 8 h (Schnoy et al., 1982; Schmidt et al., 1984). Light and electron microscopy revealed no effects on intrapulmonary nerves.

Testicular lesions, characterized by degeneration of primary spermatocytes and mild exfoliation of spermatids, were reported in a study on Sprague-Dawley rats exposed to 17 600 mg/m³ (5000 ppm) (99% pure) for 24 h (DeMartino et al., 1987). There were no deaths or other manifestations of toxicity. Complete recovery had taken place within 30 days after exposure.

8.1.2 Oral administration

Using a one-week observation period, the LD_{50} values for analytical grade *n*-hexane were estimated to be 28.7 g/kg for older adult (300-470 g) male Sprague-Dawley rats, 32.4 g/kg for young adult males (80-160 g), 15.8 g/kg for 14-day-old rats, and less than 0.7 g/kg for newborn rats (Kimura et al., 1971).

8.1.3 Dermal exposure

Signs of discomfort and incoordination, but no deaths, were noted in New Zealand male rabbits dermally exposed under an occlusive dressing for 4 h to 3 g hexane (45% *n*-hexane) per kg (Hine & Zuidema, 1970).

8.1.4 Parenteral administration

Following intraperitoneal injection of 3.6 g *n*-hexane (analytical grade) per kg, 8 out of 10 guinea-pigs died within 24 h (Wahlberg & Boman, 1979). The approximate lethal intraperitoneal doses of hexane were reported to be 530 mg/kg at an environmental temperature of 36 °C, 4000 mg/kg at 8 °C, and 9100 mg/kg at 26 °C in male and female albino Sprague-Dawley rats (Keplinger et al., 1959). All of 10 male NMRI mice died following slow intravenous infusion of *n*-hexane (purity not stated, 830 mg/kg) in a lipid emulsion. A dose of 750 mg/kg was estimated to be the ED_{50} value for loss of righting reflex (Jeppsson, 1975).

8.1.5 In vitro exposure

Gillies et al. (1980) investigated whether or not the inhibition of sterologenesis induced by chronic ingestion of 2,5-hexanedione could also be induced *in vitro*. Sterologenesis was not inhibited in sciatic nerves of rats incubated with 2,5-hexanedione (1 mmol/litre for 3 h). Although it has been shown that 2,5-hexanedione and other compounds that cause distal axonopathy inhibit cholesterol biosynthesis, Gillies et al. (1980) proposed that the neurotoxicity of 2,5-hexanedione is related to the inhibition of the biosynthesis of ubiquinone rather than that of cholesterol. Perfusion of isolated New Zealand rabbit hearts with an *n*-hexane (laboratory grade) solution of 9.6 mg/litre for 1 h reduced the force of cardiac contraction, but no effects on heart rate or coronary blood flow were reported. Histopathological examination showed shrinkage of myocardial fibres (Raje, 1983). The dose for 50% inhibition (IC_{50}) of cytochrome-P-450-dependent benzyloxy-dealkylase activity by *n*-hexane in lung microsomes from β-naphthoflavone-treated rats was found to be 8.8 ± 3.2 μmol/litre (Rabovsky & Judy, 1989).

Decreased oxygen consumption at *n*-hexane (purity not specified) plate concentrations of 40 μg/mg or more was reported following incubation (15-38 °C) of rabbit cardiac mitochondria with 0-160 μg *n*-hexane/mg mitochondrial protein (Borgatti et al., 1981). Adding 1.7 to 20 μl of *n*-hexane (pure) to a 500-μl suspension of isolated human erythrocytes resulted in a dose-dependent increase of specific binding to insulin. In the extracellular medium a simultaneous increase in the amount of degraded insulin, dependent on the concentration of *n*-hexane, was recorded. *n*-Hexane may affect the availability of membrane receptors for hormones (Svabova et al., 1987).

In studies by Notten & Henderson (1975a), male guinea-pigs were given daily ip injections of *n*-hexane (purity not specified) of 3 or 60 mg/kg per day in sesame oil for 3 days and killed on day 4. The livers were removed for homogenization, and the mitochondrial supernatant was incubated with 0.1 or 0.5% (v/v) *n*-hexane (purity not specified). With preparations from animals treated with

60 mg/kg per day, there was a dose-dependent increase in uridine 5'-diphosphate (UDP) glucuronidation of *p*-nitrophenol, and a slight decrease in *p*-hydroxylation of aniline, but no effect on *N*-demethylation of aminopyrine. There was no effect on UDP glucuronidation of *p*-nitrophenol when a guinea-pig microsomal preparation, pre-activated with Triton X-100, was used (Notten & Henderson, 1975a). In hepatic microsomal preparations (from untreated guinea-pigs) incubated with up to 7% (v/v) *n*-hexane (purity not specified) for 20 min, glucuronidation of *p*-nitrophenol and *o*-aminophenol was increased. Aniline *p*-hydroxylation was increased at *n*-hexane concentrations below 0.1%. *N*-demethylation of aminopyrine was reduced in a dose-related manner at *n*-hexane concentrations above 0.5% (Notten & Henderson, 1975b).

In male Wistar rat hepatic microsome preparations incubated with *n*-hexane (analytical grade) at concentrations of 0.44, 1.11, or 2.21 mol/litre for 15 min, there was an increase in UDP-glucuronosyl-transferase activity only at 2.21 mol/litre (Vainio, 1974). Rabovsky et al. (1986) investigated the effect of *n*-hexane (2 mmol per litre) on the activities of benzo[*a*]pyrene hydroxylase and 7-ethoxycoumarin de-ethylase in rat liver and lung microsomes. The approximate extent of enzyme inhibition was 55% and 30% in the case of benzopyrene hydroxylase and 50% and 35% in the case of 7-ethoxycoumarin de-ethylase for liver and lung, respectively. In rat hepatocytes there was a slight increase (14%) in oxygen consumption and minimal leakage of aspartate aminotransferase following incubation with *n*-hexane (20 mmol/litre) for 1 h (Berger & Sozeri, 1987). At concentrations approaching the solubility limit (about 0.08 mmol/litre), *n*-hexane selectively stimulated the slow phase of cholesterol metabolism in isolated rat adrenal mitochondria (McNamara & Jefcoate, 1988). This effect was dependent on mitochondrial integrity and is apparently due to facilitation of the transfer of cholesterol from the outer membrane to the inner membrane where the responsible enzymes reside.

8.2 Short- and long-term exposures

8.2.1 *Inhalation studies*

Combined groups of 10 weanling and 10 young adult male Fischer-344 rats were exposed to an *n*-hexane (95% pure) concentration of 3520 mg/m^3 (1000 ppm) for 24 h/day, 7 days/week, for 4 weeks and then for 24 h/day, 6 days per week, for 7 weeks. There was reduced weight gain, and 5 out of 10 adults died by week 14 (Howd et al., 1983). When the same strain of rats was exposed for 24 h/day, 5 days per week, to an *n*-hexane (95% pure) level of 3520 mg/m^3, there was inhibition of body weight gain (Pryor et al., 1982). In both studies, some recovery of body weight occurred after the end of exposure. Body weight gain was reduced in Sprague-Dawley rats, exposed for up to 6 months, 22 h/day, to an *n*-hexane (95% pure) concentration of 1760 mg/m^3 (500 ppm) (API, 1983a,b).

In Wistar rats exposed to 35 200 mg/m^3 (10 000 ppm) *n*-hexane (96-99% pure), 8 h/day, 7 days/week, for 15 or 19 weeks, there was loss of body weight and some deaths occurred (Altenkirch et al., 1978). The same results were reported for male Wistar rats exposed to 10 563 mg/m^3 (3000 ppm) *n*-hexane (99% pure) for 12 h/day, 7 days/week, for 16 weeks (Takeuchi et al., 1980). Reduced body weight gain was noted in Wistar rats exposed 12 h/day for 16 weeks to 3520 mg/m^3 (1000 ppm) *n*-hexane (99% pure) (Takeuchi et al., 1981) and in Fischer-344 male weanling rats exposed 14 h/day, 7 days/week, for 14 weeks to *n*-hexane (95% pure) (Pryor et al., 1983). A dose-related reduced weight gain was also reported in male Wistar rats exposed to 704 or 1760 mg/m^3 (200 or 500 ppm) *n*-hexane (99% pure), 12 h/day, for 24 weeks (Ono et al., 1982). No effect on body weight was noted in Sprague-Dawley rats exposed to *n*-hexane (analytical grade) (443 mg/m^3, 126 ppm), 21 h/day, 7 days/week, for up to 34 weeks (API, 1978), or in male Wistar rats exposed to 373 mg/m^3 (106 ppm) *n*-hexane, for 12 h/day, 7 days/week, for 24 weeks (Takeuchi et al., 1983). No statistically significant effects on body weight were reported in Wistar rats exposed to concentrations of 352, 1056, or 3168 mg/m^3 (100, 300, or 900 ppm) *n*-hexane (99% pure) for 8 h/day, 5 days/week, for 72 weeks (De Groot & Kepner, 1984).

8.2.1.1 Combined-exposure effects

The neuropathic effects of *n*-hexane on rats are enhanced by co-exposure to methyl ethyl ketone. Clinical signs and histological evidence of neuropathy developed earlier and were more severe in male Wistar rats exposed to *n*-hexane (31 328 mg/m^3, 8900 ppm) with methyl ethyl ketone (MEK) (3250 mg/m^3, 1100 ppm) for 8 h/day, 7 days per week, for 15 weeks, or 31 680 mg *n*-hexane/m^3 (9000 ppm) with 2950 mg MEK/m^3 (1000 ppm) for 19 weeks than in those exposed to 35 200 mg *n*-hexane/m^3 (10 000 ppm) alone (Altenkirch et al., 1978). In another study, male Wistar rats were exposed to 1760 or 2646 mg/m^3 (500 or 700 ppm) *n*-hexane (purity not specified) or *n*-hexane-MEK mixtures of 1056 mg/m^3 (300 ppm) plus 590 mg/m^3 (200 ppm), 1408 mg/m^3 (400 ppm) plus 295 mg/m^3 (100 ppm), or 1760 mg/m^3 (500 ppm) plus 590 mg/m^3 (Altenkirch et al., 1982). There was a reduction in the time to onset of hindlimb paralysis in rats exposed continuously to 1408 mg *n*-hexane/m^3 plus 295 mg MEK/m^3 compared with those exposed only to 1760 mg *n*-hexane/m^3. Hypersalivation occurred in rats exposed to the mixtures in both studies. Reduced tail motor and mixed nerve conduction velocities were reported in male Wistar rats after 20 weeks of exposure (12 h/day) to 352 mg *n*-hexane/m^3 (100 ppm) plus 590 mg MEK/m^3 (200 ppm), but there were no toxicologically significant effects with the same concentration of either chemical alone (Takeuchi et al., 1983).

Methyl isobutyl ketone (MIBK) enhances *n*-hexane-induced neurotoxicity in hens. Abou-Donia et al. (1985a) treated groups of 5 hens for 90 days with 3520 mg *n*-hexane/m^3 (1000 ppm) simultaneously with 0, 410, 1025, 2050, or 4100 mg MIBK/m^3 (0, 100, 250, 500, or 1000 ppm). An untreated control group and a group treated with MIBK (4100 mg/m^3) alone were also included. The treatments were followed by a 30-day observation period. *n*-Hexane alone produced mild ataxia, while hens exposed to mixtures of *n*-hexane and MIBK exhibited clinical signs of neurotoxicity accompanied by large swollen axons and degeneration of the axon and myelin of the spinal cord and peripheral nerves. The severity of neurotoxicity depended on the dose of the non-neurotoxic agent MIBK. The synergistic effect of MIBK may be related to its ability to induce the cytochrome P-450 system responsible for the metabolism of *n*-hexane to neurotoxic metabolites.

A marked increase in the clinical signs of impaired limb function in male Wistar rats exposed to 2464 mg/m^3

(700 ppm) *n*-hexane (purity not specified), 23 h/day for 7-9 weeks, followed pre-treatment with, and subsequent co-exposure to, lead acetate. These effects did not occur with lead acetate alone (Wagner et al., 1984).

n-Hexane-induced neurotoxicity can be reduced by co-exposure to toluene. Effects on nerve conduction were less marked when rats were exposed 12 h/day for 16 weeks to a mixture of 3696 mg/m³ (1050 ppm) *n*-hexane (99% pure) and 3940 mg toluene/m³ (1050 ppm) than when they were exposed to 3696 mg *n*-hexane/m³ alone (Takeuchi et al., 1981). On the other hand, Ikeda et al. (1986) showed that co-administration of *n*-hexane and toluene may potentiate central nervous system toxicity. Male Wistar rats were exposed to a mixture of 704 mg *n*-hexane/m³ and 750 mg toluene/m³ (200 ppm each) continuously for 30 days. The treatment produced a decrease in the dopamine levels in the midbrain and hypothalamus and an increase in the hippocampus. These changes were not found following exposure to either solvent alone.

The effects of longer exposure (22 h/day, 7 days/week, for 6 months) to mixtures of *n*-hexane (1760 mg/m³, 500 ppm) and an equal concentration of other hexane "iso-mers" (true isomers and related 6-carbon compounds) have been studied (Spencer, 1982; API, 1983a,b). The other hexane isomers appeared to have no effect on the neuro-pathic activity of *n*-hexane in rats. A similar pattern of neuropathy was seen as a result of exposure to 1760 mg *n*-hexane/m³ both with (at an equal concentration) or without other hexane "isomers". There were no neuro-pathic changes following exposure to 440 mg *n*-hexane/m³ (125 ppm) either with (at 3 or 11 times the *n*-hexane con-centration) or without other hexane "isomers". Pellin et al. (1988) investigated the possibility of an interactive effect of *n*-hexane and organophosphorus compounds on neurotoxicity. Hens that were pretreated with *n*-hexane (300 mg/kg per day ip for 7-15 days) showed a synergistic effect for the inhibition of neuropathy target esterase (NTE) and acetyl- and butyryl-cholinesterase induced by a single oral dose of tri-*o*-cresyl phosphate (TOCP). At a lower dose of TOCP (20 mg/kg), which was not neurotoxic, there was still an increase in NTE inhibition to levels close to the minimum threshold associated with neuropathy.

8.2.1.2 Effects on the respiratory tract

In studies by Dunnick (1989) and Dunnick et al. (1989), $B6C3F_1$ mice were exposed to 0, 1760, 3520, 14 080, and 35 200 mg n-hexane/m^3 (0, 500, 1000, 4000, and 10 000 ppm) for 6 h/day, 5 days/week, for 13 weeks, and also to 3520 mg/m^3 for 22 h/day, 5 days/week, for 13 weeks. Body weight gain was reduced at 35 200 mg/m^3 (6 h/day) and at 3520 mg/m^3 (22 h/day). The final mean body weights were 17% and 10% lower, respectively, for males and 6% and 0% lower, respectively, for females. Sneezing was also observed at 35 200 mg/m^3. Histopathological changes included mild inflammatory, erosive, and regenerative lesions in the olfactory and respiratory epithelium of the nasal cavity at 14 080 and 35 000 mg per ^{3} (6 h/day) and at 3520 mg/m^3 (22 h/day).

In male Wistar rats exposed to n-hexane (96-99% pure) 8 h/day, at concentrations of 1760 mg/m^3 (500 ppm) for 48-70 days, 2464 mg/m^3 (700 ppm) for 7 days, or 35 200 mg/m^3 (10 000 ppm) for 2-4 days, there were ultrastructural changes in the lungs. Light microscopy did not reveal any confirmed pathological changes in the lung tissue of animals that had been exposed over 4-24 h to n-hexane or to mixtures of n-hexane and methyl ethyl ketone (MEK). Cytoplasmic swelling and focal desquamation of alveolar epithelium followed exposure over 2-7 days to 2464-35 200 mg/m^3 (Schnoy et al., 1982). Numerous fat-laden alveolar macrophages, degenerate type 1 pneumocytes and increased numbers of alveolar brush cells occurred after 7 days of exposure to 1760 mg/m^3 (500 ppm). The basic structures of alveoli and alveolar receptors were preserved. The authors hypothesized that n-hexane alone or in combination with methyl ethyl ketone caused fatty degeneration of the alveolar epithelium due to interference with cellular metabolism. Under identical test conditions axonal changes in pulmonary nerves were reported (Schmidt et al., 1984). More pronounced effects, including degenerative changes in the ciliary cells of small air passages, followed exposure to mixtures of 1056-1760 mg n-hexane/m^3 (300-500 ppm) plus 295-590 mg MEK/m^3 (100-200 ppm) for 24-89 days or 31 680 mg n-hexane/m^3 (9000 ppm) plus 2950 mg MEK/m^3 (1000 ppm) for 2-14 days. However, no treatment-related lesions were observed in the lungs of rats (Wistar, Fischer-344, CD) exposed to *n*-hexane by a variety of exposure patterns. These included exposures to up to 35 200 mg/m^3 (10 000 ppm) over 13 weeks and 3168 mg/m^3 (900 ppm) over 72 weeks (Kurita, 1974; Toxigenics, 1982; API, 1983a,b; De Groot & Kepner, 1984).

In New Zealand rabbits, severe respiratory tract lesions followed exposures to an *n*-hexane (research grade) concentration of 10 560 mg/m^3 (3000 ppm), 8 h/day, for 8 days (Lungarella et al., 1980, 1984; Barni-Comparini et al., 1982). Centriacinar emphysema and scattered microhaemorrhages were observed, lung damage being most marked at the transition zone between the terminal bronchioles and alveolar ducts. Focal subpleural atelectasis, and alveolar and interstitial oedema were also observed. In another study (Lungarella et al., 1984), 24 New Zealand male rabbits were exposed to 10 560 mg/m^3, 8 h/day, 5 days/week, for 24 weeks. Clinical signs of ocular and upper respiratory tract irritation and difficulty in respiration were reported, but there was no evidence of neurotoxicity. Animals sacrificed 1 day after the last exposure showed inflammation of the nasal turbinates and necrotic erosion of the nasal mucosa. The lungs showed centriacinar emphysema, scattered foci of pulmonary fibrosis, and papillary proliferations of non-ciliated bronchiolar cells (described by the authors as papillary tumours). In a group of rabbits retained following the end of exposure for a further 120 days, irregular foci of cellular proliferation, papillary proliferations of non-ciliated bronchiolar epithelium, scattered pulmonary fibrosis, and centriacinar emphysema were still present.

Dose-related biochemical changes, indicative of increased pulmonary secretion and cell damage in the lungs, were reported in lung lavage fluid of male Sprague-Dawley rats exposed to *n*-hexane (purity not stated) concentrations of 1690, 4048, or 5833 mg/m^3 (480, 1150, or 1657 ppm) for 6 h/day, 5 days/week, for 4 weeks (Sahu et al., 1982). There were dose-related increases in protein, lipid, and sialic content and in acid and alkaline phosphatase, lactate dehydrogenase, glucose-6-phosphate dehydrogenase, and angiotensin-converting enzyme activities. Altered enzyme activity was reported in the lungs of New Zealand rabbits exposed to 10 560 mg *n*-hexane/m^3 (3000 ppm) 8 h/day for 8 days (Barni-Comparini et al., 1982). The activities of acid phosphatase, β-glucuronidase, lactate dehydrogenase, and glucose 6-phosphate dehydrogenase were significantly increased.

In a study by Hadjiivanova et al. (1987), male Wistar rats were treated with *n*-hexane by inhalation at a concentration of 14 995 mg/m^3 (4260 ppm, 5 h/day) and pulmonary surfactant was examined at 1 and 15 days. There was a treatment-dependent moderate increase in the phospholipids of the bronchoalveolar lavage, and an altered relative concentration of individual phospholipids in lung tissue homogenate. In combination with irradiation, *n*-hexane treatment depleted lung tissue phospholipids due to their release in the alveoli.

8.2.1.3 Effects on the testes

When Sprague-Dawley rats were exposed to 17 600 mg *n*-hexane/m^3 (5000 ppm) for 16 h/day, 6 days/week, up to the development of clear symptoms of polyneuropathy, damage to the germinal epithelium increased with increasing exposure. Early signs were abnormalities in primary spermatocytes including vacuolation of the cytoplasm and nuclear pycnosis. Maturing spermatids were also affected and showed swollen cytoplasm and multinucleated heads with vacuolation. Sertoli cells revealed vacuolation of the cytoplasm, primarily in the basal region, and retraction of the apical cytoplasm. Shedding of damaged spermatocytes and spermatids into the lumen of the tubule and their appearance in the epididymis were also reported. Progressive damage continued after cessation of dosing, leading to tubules devoid of all germinal cells, with the exception of some spermatogonia, and containing only damaged Sertoli cells. The authors could not determine whether the primary effect was on the Sertoli cell, the germinal cells, or both. Signs of testicular damage were clear before neuropathic symptoms developed in the rats (DeMartino et al., 1987).

These results are comparable to testicular effects reported after dosing orally with 2,5-hexanedione, a metabolite of *n*-hexane, which is the probable causative agent for these effects (see section 8.7). A decrease in relative testis weight was reported in adult and weanling

Fischer-344 rats 5 weeks after the end of exposure to 3520 mg/m³ (1000 ppm) *n*-hexane (95% pure), 24 h/day, 7 days per week, for 4 weeks followed by the same concentration, 24 h/day, 6 days/week, for a further 7 weeks; the testes were not examined histologically (Howd et al., 1983). No testicular lesions were reported in Wistar or CD rats exposed for up to 6 months to 1760 mg/m³ (500 ppm) or 18 months to 3168 mg/m³ (900 ppm) *n*-hexane (99% pure) (API, 1983a,b; De Groot & Kepner, 1984). There was slight congestion in the testes of Wistar rats following inhalation of 2992 mg/m³ (850 ppm) *n*-hexane (purity not specified), 6 days/week, for 20 weeks (Kurita, 1974). There were no testicular lesions in Fischer-344 rats exposed to 10 560, 22 880, or 35 200 mg/m³ (3000, 6500, or 10 000 ppm) *n*-hexane (99.5% pure), 6 h/day, 5 days/week, for 13 weeks (Toxigenics, 1982; Cavender et al., 1984). However, adult male Sprague-Dawley rats continuously exposed to *n*-hexane for 61 days at 3520 mg/m³ (1000 ppm) showed lesions of the tubule. All germinal cells were progressively lost leaving Sertoli cells (damaged) as the only component of the tubule. There was no impairment of androgen synthesis, and circulating androgen levels were not different from controls. Simultaneous administration of 3520 mg *n*-hexane/m³ with 4340 mg xylene/m³ (1000 ppm) caused no adverse effects on the testis (Nylen et al., 1989).

8.2.1.4 *Other effects*

Panlobular necrosis occurred in the livers of some male CD rats exposed to *n*-hexane (99% pure) concentrations of 440 or 1760 mg/m³ (125 or 500 ppm) 22 h/day, 7 days/week, for up to 6 months, and relative liver weight was increased at 1760 mg/m³ (API, 1983a). However, no hepatic effects were reported at 1760 mg/m³ in a further study (API, 1983b). Increased relative liver weight and increases in hepatic microsomal protein, cytochrome P-450 and cytochrome b5 levels have been reported in NMRI mice exposed to 88 000 to 105 600 mg/m³ (25 000 to 30 000 ppm) *n*-hexane (analytical grade), 23 h/day, for up to 4 days; no histological examination was performed (Krämer et al., 1974). Howd et al. (1983) found an increase in relative liver weight in Fischer-344 rats exposed to 3520 mg/m³ (1000 ppm) *n*-hexane (95% pure), 24 h/day for 4 weeks followed by 24 h/day (6 days/week) for 7 weeks.

Increased relative kidney weights were reported in two studies on male CD rats exposed to 1760 mg/m^3 (500 ppm) *n*-hexane (99% pure) continuously for up to 6 months (API, 1983a,b). In one study, there were traces of degenerative and regenerative changes in the kidneys of 4/34 exposed rats (API, 1983a), but in the other no renal lesions were reported (API, 1983b). In male Fischer-344 rats exposed to 10 560, 22 880, or 35 200 mg/m^3 (3000, 6500, or 10 000 ppm) *n*-hexane (99.5% pure), 6 h/day, 5 days/week, for 13 weeks, relative kidney weights were increased in rats exposed to 22 880 and 35 200 mg/m^3 and there was a reduction in urinary pH at 35 200 mg/m^3, but no treatment-related renal lesions were observed (Cavender et al., 1984).

A slight increase in giant cell numbers and haemosiderin precipitation was reported in the spleens of male Wistar rats exposed to 2992 mg/m^3 (850 ppm) *n*-hexane (purity not stated) continuously, 6 days/week, for 20 weeks (Kurita, 1974).

No significant haematological changes followed exposure to *n*-hexane in studies on Fischer-344, Wistar, and CD rats and New Zealand rabbits (Kurita, 1974; API, 1978; Rebert et al., 1982; Cavender et al., 1984; Lungarella et al., 1984). Slight reductions in blood haemoglobin and in red cell and total white cell counts, and an increase in immature cells in the bone marrow were reported in guinea-pigs exposed by inhalation to *n*-hexane of unstated purity (Spagna et al., 1967). Exposures were to 4928 mg/m^3 (1400 ppm), 2 h/day for 120 days, 29 920 mg/m^3 (8500 ppm), 2 h/day for 60 days, or to 149 952 mg/m^3 (42 600 ppm), 2 h/day for 30 days. The haematological effects occurred at 149 952 mg/m^3 and, to a lesser extent, at 29 920 mg/m^3 but not at 4928 mg/m^3.

In other studies on Fischer-344, Wistar, and CD rats, no treatment-related lesions were reported in the spleen (or other lymphoid organs) or salivary glands following exposures to 1760 mg/m^3 (500 ppm) for 6 months, 3168 mg/m^3 (900 ppm) for 72 weeks, or 35 200 mg/m^3 (10 000 ppm) for 13 weeks (Toxigenics, 1982; API, 1983a,b; Cavender et al., 1984; De Groot & Kepner, 1984).

In Wistar rats exposed to *n*-hexane (purity not stated) concentrations of 1760-2464 mg/m^3 (500-700 ppm),

22 h/day, 7 days/week, for up to 9 weeks, there was fatty degeneration and glandular duct widening of the parotid and salivary glands (Altenkirch et al., 1982). The effects were more noticeable in the rats exposed to mixtures of *n*-hexane and methyl ethyl ketone, and were associated with hypersalivation.

8.2.2 Oral studies

Body weight gain was reduced in male CD rats given (by gavage) *n*-hexane (99% pure) doses of 570 or 1140 mg/kg per day, 5 days/week, for 13 weeks, 4000 mg/kg per day for 17 weeks, or 4000 mg/kg per day technical grade hexane (40% *n*-hexane), 5 days/week, for 13 weeks or until hind-limb paralysis was observed. Severe hindlimb weakness or paralysis (from about day 100), tibial nerve lesions, and atrophy of testicular germinal epithethelium were reported in the rats given 4000 mg *n*-hexane/kg per day (Krasavage et al., 1980). The tibial nerve lesions (also found in one rat exposed to the technical grade hexane) included axonal swellings, adaxonal myelin infolding, and paranodal myelin retraction. A reduction in tail nerve conduction velocity was reported in male Wistar rats given daily doses of *n*-hexane (purity not stated) for 4 weeks (Ono et al., 1979). Doses of 0.5 or 1 g/kg per day in olive oil were given daily by gavage for 4 weeks and the rats were observed for a further 4 weeks. At 8 weeks both groups showed reduced motor and mixed nerve conduction velocities.

A slight reduction in body weight gain (but no clinical or pathological signs of neurotoxicity or other gross pathological effects) was reported in male CD rats given a solution (less than 1%) of commercial hexane containing 40% *n*-hexane as drinking-water for 10 months (O'Donaghue et al., 1978a; Krasavage et al., 1979).

In a toxicity study in rats, five groups of 30 male and 30 female Wistar rats each received daily doses of 0, 0.04, 0.2, 1, or 5 g commercial hexane/kg body weight by gavage for 13 weeks. Increased relative kidney weights were observed in the rats that received 0.2, 1, or 5 g/kg, and histopathological changes occurred in the kidneys of both male and female rats that received 5 g/kg. Rats given 0.2, 1, or 5 g/kg also showed increased liver weights.

Changes in plasma enzymes, indicative of liver damage and elevated cholesterol and triglyceride levels, were detected in the highest-dose group. Also in this group, histopathological changes were detected in the adrenals, liver, kidneys, peripheral nerves, spleen, testes, and thymus. It was concluded that the no-observed-effect level of technical hexane is 0.04 g/kg body weight per day but treatment-related effects at the adjacent dose level (0.2 g/kg per day) were slight and occurred in male rats only (Til et al., 1989).

8.2.3 Dermal studies

No deaths and no effects on weight gain occurred in guinea-pigs for up to one month following dermal appli-cation (sealed chamber) of 3.5 g n-hexane (analytical grade) per kg for one week (Wahlberg & Boman, 1979).

Abou-Donia et al. (1985b) investigated the neurotox-icity of n-hexane, 2,5-hexanediol, and 2,5-hexanedione in hens with and without 0-ethyl-0-4-nitrophenyl phenyl-phosphonothioate (EPN). Following a daily dermal appli-cation of n-hexane (1 mmol/kg) for 90 days followed by a 30-day observation period, leg weakness was observed. The other two aliphatic hexacarbons were more toxic at this dose level causing gross ataxia. Concurrent dermal appli-cation of EPN with n-hexane or 2,5-hexanediol at the same or different sites produced an additive neurotoxic action with histopathological changes characteristic of EPN neurotoxicity. The additive effect of n-hexane and 2,5-hexanediol and a potentiating effect of 2,5-hexanedione were considered to result from the enhancing effect of the hexacarbons on EPN absorption and/or metabolism.

8.2.4 In vitro studies

In mouse spinal cord/dorsal root ganglion/thigh-muscle explants incubated with n-hexane (97% pure), axonal swellings, degeneration of central and peripheral nerve fibre, and necrosis of muscle fibres were reported (Veronesi et al., 1983, 1984). In explants exposed to 25, 50, 80, 100, or 250 μg n-hexane/ml for up to 8 weeks, giant axonal swellings developed at 100 μg/ml or more and appeared first in distal, paranodal regions of large diameter fibres (Veronesi et al., 1984). Explants exposed to 50-650 µg/ml for 3-8 weeks showed marked changes in nerve fibres at 400-650 µg/ml after 4-5 days and progressive axonal changes at 245-325 µg/ml after 2-6 weeks (Veronesi et al., 1983). In this study, explants removed from exposure and maintained in plain nutrient solution for 12-15 weeks showed some remyelination of viable axons. Exposure of explants to *n*-hexane with non-cytotoxic levels of methyl ethyl ketone potentiated the axonal effects. Cytoplasmic bubbling and lysosome proliferation were reported in murine neuroblastoma cells incubated with up to 1.5% *n*-hexane (purity not stated) for up to 10 days (Selkoe et al., 1978).

8.2.5 Parenteral studies

n-Hexane administered subcutaneously to mice at doses of up to 10 ml/kg was found to decrease metallothionein concentrations in the pancreas. The maximum effect was observed 24 h after administration. Levels had returned to normal 48 h after administration (Onosaka et al., 1988).

In male Donryu rats given subcutaneous *n*-hexane (97% pure) injections of 330 mg/kg per day, 5 days/week, for 21 weeks, there was reduced growth rate, reduced movement, disturbed gait, and decreased amplitude of the tail nerve action potential, but no effect on nerve conduction velocity (Misumi & Nagano, 1984). In male Donryu rats injected subcutaneously with *n*-hexane (purity not stated; 330 mg/kg per day, 5 days/week, for 5 months), gait disturbances and decreased sweating response to β-methylcholine were reported in all animals (Abe et al., 1980). Peripheral nerve lesions were reported in Sprague-Dawley rats following subcutaneous injections of *n*-hexane (99% pure) (650-2000 mg/kg per day, 5 days/week) for up to 35 weeks (Schaumburg & Spencer, 1976). In male Sprague-Dawley rats given daily intraperitoneal injections of *n*-hexane (purity not stated; 540 mg/kg for 5 weeks), reductions in peak conduction velocity and duration of action potentials in the sciatic and sural nerves, in the absence of any behavioural or histological effects, were reported (Anderson & Dunham, 1984).

The potential for *n*-hexane to affect the haemopoietic system was indicated by the significant inhibition of uptake of iron by the bone marrow in rats that had received

1 ml *n*-hexane/kg (ip) on two successive days (Goel et al., 1987). The effects of the metabolite 2,5-hexanediol on the spleen are discussed in section 8.7.

Hepatic necrosis occurred in male rats (strain not specified) following intraperitoneal *n*-hexane (analytical grade) injections of 660 mg/kg per day daily for 2 or 7 days or twice weekly for 45 days (Goel et al., 1982). The activities of serum acetylcholinesterase and carboxyesterase and serum levels of protein, albumin, and cholesterol were reduced in all groups.

When female albino rats were treated with *n*-hexane (1 ml/kg by intraperitoneal injection) for 1, 2, 7, and 45 days, hepatoxicity was evident from a loss of total hepatic sulfhydryl content and there was a significant increase in lipid peroxidation at 1 and 2 days. There was also a decrease in microsomal drug-metabolizing activity and microsomal glucose-6-phosphatase activity (Goel et al., 1988).

Sclerodermatous skin changes were observed in *ddy* mice after 17 daily intraperitoneal injections of 3.3 mg *n*-hexane in 1 ml of 0.9% saline (Yamakage & Ishikawa, 1982). The purity of the *n*-hexane was not stated and sclerotic skin changes also occurred in positive control mice.

Severe lung lesions, including oedema, cellular infiltration, abcesses, necrosis, fibrosis, and haemorrhage, were reported in male rabbits given daily intramuscular *n*-hexane (purity not stated) injections of 660 mg/kg undiluted for 5 days or 66 mg/kg in olive oil for 21-77 days (Taira, 1975).

Klimes et al. (1987) investigated the effect of intraperitoneal injections of *n*-hexane (1 ml/kg daily for 7 days) on the enzymic degradation of insulin. Insulin degradation in the liver of treated male Wistar rats was greater than in control rat liver. However, there was inhibition of insulin degradation in the erythrocytes of treated rats. There was, therefore, evidence for some potential disturbance by *n*-hexane of glucose tolerance. Five daily intraperitoneal doses of *n*-hexane (1 g/kg) per week for 2 weeks to female Sprague-Dawley rats (a dose equivalent to one tenth of the intraperitoneal LD_{50}) had no effect on kidney tubular function as shown by measurements of urinary N-acetyl-β-D-glucosaminidase (NAG), β_2-microglobulin and albumin (Bernard et al., 1989).

8.3 Reproduction, embryotoxicity, and teratogenicity

8.3.1 Teratogenicity studies

8.3.1.1 Inhalation studies

The exposure of groups of 7-9 pregnant Fischer-344 rats to 3520 mg/m³ (1000 ppm) n-hexane (purity unspecified) for 6 h/day on days 8-12, 12-16, or 8-16 of gestation did not result in a significant increase in resorption rate or in the incidence of visceral or skeletal malformations (Bus & Tyl, 1979; Bus et al., 1979). There were slight, but not statistically significant, increases in minor anomalies such as dilated renal pelvis and misaligned fourth sternebra in the offspring of all the exposure groups. No signs of maternal toxicity were reported. Groups of 17-20 pregnant CD rats were exposed to 327 or 1436 mg/m³ (93 or 408 ppm) n-hexane (purity not stated) for 6 h/day on days 6-15 of gestation (Litton Bionetics, 1979). There was no embryotoxicity or increase in the incidence of malformations, but small, not statistically significant, increases in the incidence of subcutaneous haematomas and retarded bone ossification were observed at both exposure levels.

A group of 14 pregnant Fischer-344 rats was exposed to 3520 mg/m³ (1000 ppm) n-hexane (99% pure) for 6 h/day on days 8-16 of gestation and allowed to deliver naturally on day 23 (Bus & Tyl, 1979; Bus et al., 1979). Litters were culled to 6 pups/litter and postnatal development was followed for 7 weeks with weaning at 4 weeks. There was no statistically significant difference between the mean litter weights of the exposed and control groups. However, a significant transient depression in mean litter weight occurred over the first 6 weeks and was most marked at week 3. There were no signs of neuropathy in the pups during the 7 weeks of observation.

In a study on the offspring of Sprague-Dawley rats exposed to 352, 7040, or 35 200 mg n-hexane/m³ (100, 2000, or 10 000 ppm), 7 h/day, from 15 days prior to conception to day 18 of gestation, no physical malformations or effects on postnatal growth rate or age at eye opening were reported (Howell, 1979; Howell & Cooper, 1981). Electrophysiological measurements of visual evoked response (VER) and inter-hemisphere evoked response (IHR) were performed on neonatal Sprague-Dawley rats from dams exposed to 0, 352, 7040, or 35 200 mg/m^3 (0, 100, 2000, or 10 000 ppm) n-hexane (purity unknown), 7 h/day, from 15 days prior to conception to day 18 of gestation (Howell, 1979; Howell & Cooper, 1981). There were no abnormalities in the VER and IHR at 11, 20, and 60 days. A significant increase in the amplitude of the early VER peaks was observed in unanaesthetized pups aged 45 days that had been exposed *in utero* to 35 200 mg/m^3. However, neither of the studies was reported in sufficient detail for an assessment of the significance of these observations to be made.

Exposure of pregnant rats (number and strain not specified) to 1760, 2815, or 5280 mg/m^3 (500, 800, or 1500 ppm) n-hexane (purity not stated) during gestation and lactation resulted in reduced maternal weight gain, increased resorption rates, reduced pup weight gain, and retardation of cerebellar histogenesis and neuronal maturation (Stoltenburg-Didinger et al., 1984). Peripheral neuropathy (motor weakness) was reported in the dams but not in the pups. Similar results were obtained following exposure to a mixture of 5280 mg n-hexane/m^3 and 4425 mg MEK/m^3 (1500 ppm) or to MEK alone at concentrations of 2360 (800 ppm) and 4425 mg/m^3.

8.3.1.2 Oral

In a study on CD 1 mice, dams were dosed with n-hexane (99% pure) at 0 (37 mice), 260 (13 mice), 660 (6 mice), 1320 (6 mice), or 2200 (14 mice) mg/kg per day (in three divided doses) on days 6-15 of gestation and killed on day 18. There were no embryotoxic, fetotoxic, or teratogenic effects. At the highest dose, one dam died, and decreased weight gain was noted in surviving dams. In a follow-up study, dams were dosed with 0 (24 mice), 2170 (24 mice), 2830 (25 mice), 7920 (34 mice), or 9900 (33 mice) mg/kg per day on days 6-15 of gestation and killed on day 18. A dose-related increase in maternal mortality was noted at daily doses of 2830 mg/kg or more. A stat-istically significant reduction in fetal weight was reported at daily doses of 7920 mg/kg or more. There were no increases in the number of resorptions or statistically significant dose-related increases in malformations (Marks et al., 1980).

8.3.2 Fertility studies

There was no reduction in male or female fertility in a dominant lethal study in which groups of 12 male CD-1 mice were exposed by inhalation to 352 or 1408 mg/m³ (100 or 400 ppm) *n*-hexane (purity unstated), 6 h/day, 5 days per week, for 8 weeks and mated during the 2 weeks follow-ing exposure (Litton Bionetics, 1980).

8.4 Mutagenicity and related end-points

n-Hexane (> 99% pure) at concentrations of up to 100 μg/plate was negative, both with and without meta-bolic activation (S-9 from the liver of rats and hamsters pretreated with Aroclor®) in a pre-incubation method using 95% ethanol as solvent and Salmonella typhimurium strains TA1535, TA1537, TA100, and TA98 (Mortelmans et al., 1986). An *n*-hexane preparation in dimethyl sulfoxide was not mutagenic in S. typhimurium strains TA92, TA94, TA98, TA100, TA1535, and TA1537 either in the presence or absence of liver S-9 fractions prepared from rats pre-treated with Kanechlor KC-400® (Ishidate & Sofuni, 1984). No evidence of mutagenic activity was reported in a microsuspension fluctuation assay with S. typhimurium (McCarroll et al., 1980).

There was no evidence of mutagenic activity using *n*-hexane (ultraviolet grade) in dimethyl sulfoxide in a TK +/- mouse lymphoma(L 5178Y) forward mutation assay with plate concentrations ranging from 80-200 μg/ml without S-9 fraction or 10-240 μg/ml in the presence or absence of metabolic activation with rat liver (Arochlor® pre-treated) S-9 fraction (Hazelton Laboratories, 1981). There were problems of cytotoxicity and possible losses of *n*-hexane by evaporation. A preliminary study using ethyl acetate as the solvent and plate concentrations of *n*-hexane (purity not specified) of 400-3200 μg per ml (without S-9 fraction) or 200-1000 μg/ml (with S-9 fraction) was inconclusive. In an automated adaptation of the S. typhimurium assay using strains TA98 and TA100, *n*-hexane was found not to be mutagenic either with or without the addition of liver S-9 fraction (Houk et al., 1989).

Lankas et al. (1978) conducted a limited investigation of the effect of *n*-hexane (certified grade) on forward mutation to ouabain resistance by Chinese hamster V79 cells at a plate concentration of 10.34 mg/litre in acetone for 2 weeks. Although a negative result was reported in this study, only one concentration was tested without exogenous metabolic activation.

Evidence of chromosomal damage following incubation with undiluted *n*-hexane (95% pure) at plate concentrations of 66, 198, or 330 μg/ml for 24 or 48 h was reported in *in vitro* studies using a Chinese hamster fibroblast cell line (CHL) without exogenous metabolic activation (Ishidate & Sofuni, 1984). An increase in polyploidy, but with no increase in structural aberrations, was noted after incubation of the cells with undiluted *n*-hexane (95% pure) at a concentration of 330 μg/ml for 48 h.

In CD rats exposed to 528, 1056, or 1805 mg/m^3 (150, 300, or 600 ppm) *n*-hexane (ultraviolet grade) vapour (6 h/day for 5 consecutive days), there was an increase in the incidence of bone marrow cells with chromatid breaks at 528 and 1056 mg/m^3 (Hazelton Laboratories, 1981). Severe chromosomal damage with fragments and dicentrics was reported at 2112 mg/m^3 (600 ppm). In a preliminary study using a different batch of *n*-hexane, an increase in the number of aberrations per cell was reported following exposure to 352 and 1408 mg/m^3 (100 and 400 ppm).

In a study on the frequency of chromosomal alterations induced in *Vicia faba* root tip cells exposed to *n*-hexane solutions in water at concentrations of 0.10, 0.30, 0.50, 0.75, and 1%, an increase in chromosomal aberrations occurred at the concentration of 0.75% but not at the other concentrations tested (Gomez-Arroyo et al., 1986).

In male Sprague-Dawley rats exposed to 17 600 mg/m^3 (5000 ppm) *n*-hexane vapour (99% pure) (16 h/day, 6 days per week), chromosomal changes were observed in the germ cells (DeMartino et al., 1987). After 2-4 weeks of exposure, spermatocytes showed an abnormal arrangement of chromosomes at metaphase and chromosomal bridges at anaphase. Spermatids had giant nuclei, probably polyploid. There was no evidence of dominant lethality when male CD-1 mice were exposed by inhalation to 352 or 1408 mg/m^3 (100 or 400 ppm) *n*-hexane (purity not stated) (6 h/day, 5 days per week for 8 weeks) and mated during the 2 weeks following exposure (Litton Bionetics, 1980). There were no effects on the number of implantations or on the dead implant/live implant ratio.

In studies by McCarroll et al. (1981a,b), microsuspension (sealed microwells for 8 h) differential toxicity assays were carried out using two bacterial species with exposure to *n*-hexane (high technical grade) in the presence and absence of Arochlor®-induced rat liver S-9. The findings were negative in at least three separate trials per strain, using *Escherichia coli* WP2, its DNA repair-deficient derivatives (WP2 uvr A, CM611, WP67, WP100, and WP110), its DNA repair-deficient derivative p3478, *Bacillus subtilis* H17, and its DNA repair-deficient derivative M45 (rec assay). The *B. subtilis* rec assay was negative for *n*-hexane both in the presence and absence of S-9 exogenous metabolic activation (Kawachi et al., 1982). There was no increase in unscheduled DNA synthesis in human lymphocytes exposed to *n*-hexane (99% pure) in 1% dimethylsulfoxide (0.008, 0.08, and 0.8 mg/ml culture) *in vitro* either with or without metabolic activation with rat liver S-9 mix. Cytotoxicity was reported at 0.08 and 0.8 mg/ml without S-9 mix (Perocco et al., 1983).

8.5 Carcinogenicity

8.5.1 Inhalation studies

In a 24-week study in which male New Zealand rabbits were exposed to an *n*-hexane (research grade) concentration of 10 560 mg/m^3 (3000 ppm) for 8 h/day, 6 days per week, papillary proliferations of non-ciliated bronchiolar cells were reported (Lungarella et al., 1984) (see section 8.2.1.2). The short duration, single exposure concentration, and the use of rabbits of only one sex present problems in interpreting this as a carcinogenicity study.

8.5.2 *Skin-painting studies*

No tumours were found in 15 C17 inbred mice following daily skin painting with *n*-hexane (solvent grade) and once-weekly application (presumably for the life-time of each animal) of croton oil (3% in liquid paraffin) as co-carcinogen (Ranadive et al., 1972).

In a tumour promotion study, 30 female mice were given a non-carcinogenic dermal dose of 7,12-dimethylbenz[*a*]-anthracene followed by a dermal application of about 20 μl *n*-hexane (99.8% pure) in cyclohexane (20 g in 100 ml) three times a week for 60 weeks (Sice, 1966). No skin tumours were reported but there was dermal irritation. A similar study using 1-hexanol (97% pure), a metabolite of *n*-hexane, and a group of 50 mice yielded similar results. However, Bock & Chortyk (1970) found that *n*-hexane induced tumours in mice previously primed with 7,12-dimethylbenz[*a*]anthracene.

8.6 Neurotoxicity

Although effects on the central nervous system have been noted, the principal toxic effect of *n*-hexane is a peripheral neuropathy.

8.6.1 *Central nervous system effects*

Altered latency and amplitude values for the fifth component of the brainstem auditory-evoked response (BAER), which reflects central nervous system activity, were reported from week 3-4 of exposure, and the visual-evoked cortical response was affected (Rebert & Sorenson, 1983). At 1760 mg/m^3 (500 ppm) (the lowest concentration investigated in this series of studies), reduced forelimb and hindlimb grip strengths and increased latency of the fifth BAER component were noted after 4-6 weeks of exposure. There was slight recovery of the amplitude of the fifth BAER component at the time of last measurement (15 weeks post exposure).

Neuropathological changes were seen in the spinal cord, medulla oblongata, and cerebellar vermis of Sprague-Dawley rats exposed for 1-23 weeks to 1408-2112 mg/m^3 (400-600 ppm) *n*-hexane (95% pure) (Spencer & Schaumburg, 1977a,b).

3

In Fischer-344 rats exposed to 10 560, 22 880, or 35 200 mg/m³ (3000, 6500, or 10 000 ppm) *n*-hexane (99.5% pure) 6 h/day, 5 days/week, for 13 weeks, axonal swelling was noted in the brain (medulla) in one out of 10 animals exposed to 35 200 mg/m³ (Cavender et al., 1984). There were no clinical signs of neurotoxicity.

8.6.2 Peripheral nervous system effects

8.6.2.1 Clinical and morphological findings

The initial clinical signs of *n*-hexane-induced neuropathy in rats are effects on the hind feet (flat foot, foot eversion), followed by a waddling gait, an inability to extend the hindlimbs, and symmetrical, distal hindlimb weakness. In the studies of Dunnick (1989) and Dunnick et al. (1989) reported in section 8.2.1.2, B6C3F mice were exposed to 0, 1760, 3520, 14 080, and 35 200 mg/m³ (0, 500, 1000, 4000, and 10 000 ppm) *n*-hexane for 6 h/day, 5 days/week, for 13 weeks. Mice were also exposed to 3520 mg/m³ for 22 h/day, 5 days/week for 13 weeks. A decrease in locomotor activity in female mice exposed to 3520 mg/m³ for 22 h/day or to 35 200 mg/m³ for 6 h/day was the only neurobehavioural effect observed. Paranodal axonal swellings in tibial nerves were observed in 3 out of 4 males and 3 out of 4 females at these concentrations, but in none of the 4 controls. The severity of the peripheral nerve lesion was mild and neither segmental demyelination nor distal axonal degeneration was observed (Dunnick, 1989; Dunnick et al., 1989). The relative insensitivity of the mouse to α-diketone neurotoxicity has been related to the relatively short length and smaller diameter of the myelinated axons in this species compared to rats or human beings (Graham & Gottfreid, 1984). There can be progression to flaccid paralysis of the hindlimbs and eventual quadriplegia (Spencer & Schaumburg, 1977b; Altenkirch et al., 1978, 1982; Howd et al., 1983).

Inhalation exposure of Sprague-Dawley rats for 1-23 weeks to *n*-hexane (98% pure) at 1408-2112 mg/m³ (400-600 ppm) produced axonal swellings, containing numerous neurofilaments, on the peripheral and central nervous systems (Schaumburg & Spencer, 1976; Spencer & Schaumburg, 1977a,b; Spencer, 1982). In limb nerves, these lesions occurred principally in long, large-diameter myelinated fibres, but were also found in smaller myelinated and unmyelinated fibres. The swellings in myelinated fibres were accompanied by paranodal myelin retraction and finally distal axon disintegration and axon loss. Remyelination and, rarely, axonal regeneration have been observed in the limb nerves of rats continuously exposed to 1408-2112 mg *n*-hexane/m^3, but the extent to which regeneration may occur post exposure *in vivo* has not been reported (Spencer & Schaumburg, 1977a). In male Sprague-Dawley rats exposed to *n*-hexane (99% pure), axonal degeneration in the tibial nerve was observed following exposure to 8800 mg/m^3 (2500 ppm) for 30 weeks or 17 600 mg/m^3 (5000 ppm) for 14 weeks (Frontali et al., 1981).

Neuropathological lesions have been reported in Sprague-Dawley rats following exposure to *n*-hexane concentrations ranging between 1408-3520 mg/m^3 (400-1000 ppm) (Schaumburg & Spencer, 1976; Spencer & Schaumburg, 1977a,b; Altenkirch et al., 1982; Pryor et al., 1982; Spencer, 1982; API, 1983a,b). Axonal swellings were observed in hindlimb nerves (tibial nerve branches to the calf and then plantar nerve branches) and in the central nervous system (spinal cord, medulla oblongata, and cerebellar vermis) of Sprague-Dawley rats exposed for 1-23 weeks to 1408-2112 mg/m^3 (400-600 ppm) *n*-hexane (98.98% pure) (Spencer & Schaumberg, 1977a,b). These occurred before the appearance of hindlimb weakness. In male CD rats exposed to 440 or 1760 mg/m^3 (125 or 500 ppm) *n*-hexane (99% pure) 22 h/day, 7 days/week, axonal swelling was seen in the tibial nerve and brain (medulla oblongata) after 2 months of exposure to 1760 mg/m^3 (Spencer, 1982; API, 1983a,b). Pronounced degeneration and loss of axons in tibial (most severe) and sciatic nerves, lumbar spinal cord, and medulla oblongata were seen after 6 months.

There was complete recovery from the effects seen at 1760 mg/m^3 (500 ppm) by 6 weeks after the end of the exposure period. Clinical signs of hindlimb paralysis had disappeared by 22 weeks after exposure to 3520 mg/m^3 (1000 ppm), but there was only partial recovery of hindlimb grip strength and slight recovery of latency of tail nerve action potential.

In male Fischer-344 rats exposed by inhalation to 3520 mg/m^3 (1000 ppm) *n*-hexane (95% pure) for 24 h/day, 5 days/week, for 11 weeks, spontaneous motor activity was inhibited (Pryor et al., 1982). Hindlimb grip strength was diminished but there was less effect on forelimb grip strength. Multisensory conditioned avoidance response and pole-climbing ability decreased after 8 weeks of exposure but recovered between weeks 18 and 36. The fifth component of the BAER showed increased latency and decreased amplitude after 3 weeks. Latency returned to normal 15 weeks after the end of exposure, although there was only a slight recovery of amplitude.

Clinical signs of chronic neurotoxicity were observed after 10 weeks in male Wistar rats exposed to 10 560 mg per m^3 (3000 ppm) *n*-hexane (99% pure) for 12 h/day, 7 days/week, for 16 weeks (Takeuchi et al., 1980). Following daily inhalation of 3696 mg/m^3 (1050 ppm) *n*-hexane (99% pure) for 16 weeks (12 h/day), tail nerve conduction velocity in male Wistar rats was reduced, but without definite clinical signs of neurotoxicity (Takeuchi et al., 1981). In another study at *n*-hexane concentrations of 722 or 1725 mg/m^3 (205 or 490 ppm) for 24 weeks there were similar findings (Ono et al., 1982). The effect was still marked 4 weeks after the end of the 16-week exposure (Takeuchi et al., 1981). Axonal swelling and demyelination were observed in the tail nerves after 24 weeks of exposure to 722 mg/m^3 (Ono et al., 1982). There were no significant effects on tail nerve conduction time in rats exposed to 373 mg/m^3 (106 ppm), 12 h/day, 7 days/week, for 24 weeks; the tail nerve of the one rat examined histologically was normal (Takeuchi et al., 1983).

Higher no-observed-effect levels have been reported for male Wistar rats in studies using daily 8-h exposures to *n*-hexane. No effects on tail nerve structure or function were observed after 33 weeks of exposure to 1795 mg/m^3 (510 ppm) *n*-hexane (97% pure) (Iwata et al., 1984). There were no clinical signs of neurotoxicity or treatment-related lesions in regions of the nervous system considered to be vulnerable to hexacarbon intoxication (including areas of the lumbar spinal cord and tibial nerve) following inhalation of 1760 or 2464 mg/m^3 (500 or 700 ppm) *n*-hexane (purity not stated) for 9 or 40 weeks (Altenkirch et al., 1982).

No clinical or histological evidence of *n*-hexane-induced peripheral or central neurotoxicity was noted in two separate studies following exposure of rats to 440 mg/m³ (125 ppm) for about 22 h/day, 7 days/week, for 26-34 weeks (API, 1978, 1983a,b; Spencer, 1981, 1982).

8.6.2.2 *Electrophysiological effects*

The behavioural and neurophysiological effects of *n*-hexane have been studied in rats exposed for 24 h/day, 5-7 days/week, for 7-11 weeks (Pryor et al., 1982; Rebert et al., 1982; Howd et al., 1983; Rebert & Sorenson, 1983). In male Fischer-344 rats, exposed by inhalation for 24 h/day, 5 days/week, for 10 or 11 weeks to 1760, 3520, or 5280 mg/m³ (500, 1000, or 1500 ppm) *n*-hexane (95% pure), clinical signs of neuropathy, impairment of a conditioned avoidance response, and increased latency in the action potential of the caudal nerve were noted at the two highest exposure levels. Grip strength was reduced in the hindlimbs and, to a lesser extent, in the forelimbs of all exposed groups (Rebert & Sorenson, 1983).

Weanling male Fischer-344 rats exposed 14 h/day, 7 days/week, for 14 weeks to 7040 mg/m³ (2000 ppm) *n*-hexane (95% pure) showed behavioural and neurophysiological effects, including reduction of motor activity, startle response, pole-climbing ability, avoidance response, and grip strength, from week 2 of treatment (Pryor et al., 1983). Tail nerve latency was prolonged from week 8, the visual evoked cortical response was increased at 6 weeks, and there was a reduced amplitude of the fifth BAER component from week 10. There was no recovery of the tail nerve latency or the fifth BAER component six weeks after exposure. The visual-evoked cortical response had fully recovered 1 week after the end of exposure.

In a study of effects on the peripheral and central nervous systems, no significant behavioural or neuropathological effects were observed in Wistar rats exposed to 352, 1056, or 3168 mg/m³ (100, 300, or 900 ppm) *n*-hexane (99% pure) for 8 h/day, 5 days/week, for 72 weeks (De Groot & Kepner, 1984). Adult male rats were exposed to 17 600 mg/m³ (5000 ppm) for 16 h/day, 6 days/week, for 4 weeks. At all weekly intervals motor conduction velocity was reduced in tail nerves and did not approach control values in a 4-week post-treatment period. Raised plasma acetycholinesterase levels (25-40%) were measured at all weekly intervals during treatment, but these returned to control values 2 weeks after the treatment (Bastone et al., 1987).

Exposure to commercial grade hexane (65-70% *n*-hexane) at concentrations of 348, 950, 1936, 3626, and 6688 mg per/m³ (99, 270, 550, 1030, and 1900 ppm), for 24 h/day, 6 days/week, for one year, caused electromyographic effects on the hindlimb muscles of male SM-A mice (Miyagaki, 1967). The effects were indicative of damage to the peripheral nervous system and included insertion-type fibrillation and polyphasic discharges at 950 mg/m³ (270 ppm) or more, spontaneous fibrillation at 3626 and 6688 mg per/m³, and reduced interference patterns at 1936 mg per m³ or more. The minor effect at 348 mg/m³ (mild polyphasic discharges) was not considered to be toxicologically significant, and 348 mg/m³ was taken as the no-observed-adverse-effect level in this study.

8.6.2.3 *Grip strength*

In male Sprague-Dawley rats exposed to *n*-hexane (99% pure) for 6-9 h/day, 5 days/week, at concentrations of 1740, 5280, 8800, or 17 600 mg/m³ (500, 1500, 2500, or 5000 ppm) for 14-30 weeks, lesions were observed in the hindlimb nerves following inhalation of 8800 or 17 600 mg/m³ (Frontali et al., 1981). In a study using repeated 10-min exposures (6-24 exposures/day, 5 days/week), reduced grip strength was noted in male Fischer-344 rats after 5-6 weeks of exposure at *n*-hexane (95% pure) levels of 84 480 to 168 960 mg/m³ (24 000 to 48 000 ppm) (Pryor et al., 1982). Amplitude and latency of the fifth BAER component were affected by exposure to 168 960 mg/m³. The amplitude decreased from week 11, and there was no recovery after the end of exposure. There were significant effects on grip strength and nerve conduction velocity in Wistar rats after exposure for 8 h/day, 5 days/week, for 8 weeks to 3168 mg hexane/m³ (900 ppm) (De Groot & Kepner, 1984).

8.7 Toxicity of *n*-hexane metabolites

The production of testicular lesions in rats following exposure to 2,5-hexanedione and other metabolites of *n*-hexane has been described by Katz et al. (1980), Krasavage et al. (1980), Cavanagh & Bennetts (1981), Chapin et al. (1982), Anthony et al. (1983), and Sayre et al. (1986). Studies in Fischer-344 rats given a 1% solution of 2,5-hexanedione in drinking-water, in which severe seminiferous epithelial degeneration and azoospermia were reported, indicated that the Sertoli cell was probably the initial target for 2,5-hexanedione action (Chapin et al., 1982, 1983). Testicular atrophy, induced by 2,5-hexanedione at levels of 0.5% and 1% in the drinking-water or 200 mg/kg per day intraperitoneally, was observed in Sprague-Dawley rats before clinical signs of neuropathy or histological axonal swelling (O'Donoghue et al., 1978b).

In Charles River CD rats treated with 1% 2,5-hexanedione in the drinking-water for 4 weeks, testicular toxicity, as shown by decreased testis weight compared to controls, and enlarged and more numerous membrane-bound vacuoles basally located in Sertoli cells, was seen, together with occasional giant cells and chromatin margination in spermatids. Brain and testis tubulin from treated animals was found to be cross-linked and had a shortened nucleation phase of assembly and a more rapid rate of elongation. Tubulin cross-linking was postulated to play an important role in the testicular toxicity of the γ-diketone (Boekelheide, 1987). When Boekelheide (1988a) treated Charles River CD rats intraperitoneally with 4 mmol 2,5-hexanedione/kg per day, 5 days/week, for 2 weeks, no evidence of neurotoxicity was seen. Testis weight and histology were normal 2 weeks after the start of dosing, but large basally located Sertoli cell vacuoles were seen in the testis at 4 weeks. At 7 weeks most of the seminiferous tubules were normal and vacuolation of Sertoli cells was no longer prominent. In the same study, rats were treated with 1% 2,5-hexanedione in the drinking-water for 2 or 3 weeks. Only after 3 weeks was neurotoxicity evident from an unsteady gait. Decreased testicular weights were observed 7 weeks from the start of dosing in both groups, and loss of germ cells in seminiferous tubules was seen in both groups. At 27 weeks the testis weights were variable with partial recovery to normal values, and there was variable repopulation of seminiferous tubules. Rats were also dosed with 1% 2,5-hexanedione in the drinking-water for 5 weeks. This produced moderate to severe clinical neurotoxicity, and basally located vacuoles first appeared in Sertoli cells at 4 weeks. There was progressive necrosis and generalized sloughing of germ cells. A 17-week recovery period resulted in an absence of all postspermatogonial germ cells from the seminiferous epithelium in 3 out of 5 treated rats (Boekelheide 1988a). Under identical conditions of treatment and recovery, pyrrole reactivity of testis proteins increased to maximal levels within 2 weeks of treatment and nucleation time for microtubule assembly from purified testis tubulin was decreased at 2 weeks. This was associated with the presence of cross-linked tubulin, which was suggested to lead to germ cell loss (Boekelheide, 1988b).

In a study by Boekelheide & Eveleth (1988), Charles River CD rats were treated with a total dose of 131 (± 2) mmol 2,5-hexanedione/kg at dose rates ranging from 1.9 to 6.1 mmol/kg per day, and testicular damage was assessed 4 weeks after the cessation of treatment. Reduced testis weight and germ cell depletion were dependent on the rate of intoxication rather than the total dose. The rate of intoxication also determined the extent of testis pyrrole formation.

The metabolite 2,5-hexanediol was found to have an effect on the spleens of female albino rats (Goel et al., 1987). Following oral dosing with 2,5-hexanediol (960 mg/kg) daily for 7 days, the haematocrit value, haemoglobin content, and level of neutrophils were raised, while the level of lymphocytes was reduced relative to controls. The same treatment led to a significantly greater uptake of iron into the spleen and a significant inhibition of spleen δ-aminolevulinic acid dehydratase activity.

Atrophy of the spleen, thymus, and lymph nodes has been reported in albino rats given oral doses of 0.25, 0.5, 0.75, or 1 ml 2,5-hexanedione/kg body weight (Singh et al., 1983, 1984; Kannan et al., 1985). Atrophy of the thymus, due to loss of cortical cells, was severe but reversible. Immunocompetence (including resistance to endotoxin shock) was impaired in mice. Lymphoid lesions have been reported in rats dosed orally with 2,5-hexanedione (0.428 ml/kg) (Upreti et al., 1986).

2,5-Hexanedione is thought to be the ultimate neurotoxic metabolite of *n*-hexane (Graham et al., 1982a). An intermediate metabolite, 2,5-hexanediol, has been found to produce widespread axonal swellings throughout the nervous system including severe swelling in the distal optic tract (Cavanagh & Bennetts, 1981). Axonal swellings did not progress and were reversible (Cavanagh, 1982; Jones & Cavanagh, 1982). However, there was progression to axonal degeneration during and/or after exposure in long, large-diameter fibres of hindlimb nerves and many spinal tracts. No significant regeneration of peripheral nerves was seen. In a study on cats exposed to 2-hexanone, one animal, retained for 4½ months after exposure ceased, still showed a moderate loss of myelinated nerve fibres and axonal degeneration in the sciatic nerve (Saida et al., 1976). Using a sensitive automated technique for detecting altered coordination of hindlimb movement in male Wistar rats, Kulig et al. (1985) detected impairment of coordination 1 week after oral treatment with 600 mg 2,5-hexanedione/kg and 2 weeks after treatment with 250 mg/kg. The performance of the rats treated with 600 mg/kg was still impaired relative to controls 5 weeks after treatment. In the optic tract of cats, 2,5-hexanedione (given as a 0.5% solution in drinking-water up to a cumulative maximum of 5.8 ml/kg; maximum of 62 days of dosing) caused axonal swellings that were not selective for fibre size, impaired axonal transport, and neuronal degeneration in large cells. There was also a loss of flicker resolution (Pasternak et al., 1985).

Reduced glucose utilization and altered blood flow and glucose uptake in various areas of the brain have been reported in rats exposed to 2,5-hexanedione (Griffiths et al., 1981; Cooper et al., 1985). The inferior colliculus was one of the regions most affected in terms of reduced glucose utilization. This region is believed to be the site where the fifth component of the brainstem auditory evoked response (BAER) is generated and this component has been shown to be affected in rats by *n*-hexane exposure (Rebert et al., 1982; Pryor et al., 1982, 1983; Howd et al., 1983; Rebert & Sorenson, 1983). Oral treatment of male Sprague-Dawley rats with 2,5-hexanedione (1% in drinking-water) led to increased plasma concentrations of acetylcholinesterase at 2 and 4 weeks ($p < 0.05$ and

< 0.01, respectively). This agrees with the observed increase of plasma acetylcholinesterase following *n*-hexane inhalation (section 8.6).

Graham et al. (1982a) suggested that the accumulation of neurofilaments is not secondary to a defect in axonal transport that may be brought about by impairment of energy production by 2-hexanone or 2,5-hexanedione (Sabri et al., 1979; Sabri, 1984), but rather that the aggregation may be a primary event leading to altered axonal transport. 2,5-Hexanedione-induced neurofilament cross-linking was proposed as a mechanism leading to occlusion of flow at the nodes of Ranvier, with subsequent enlargement of the axon proximal and degenerative changes distal to this point (Graham et al., 1982b). Polymer formation by cross-linking of nerve protein (see section 6.1.3) was demonstrated using an analogue of 2,5-hexanedione (3,5-dimethyl-2,5-hexanedione) which underwent pyrrole formation more rapidly (Graham et al., 1985).

DeCaprio & O'Neill (1985) treated male Wistar rats with 0.5% 2,5-hexanedione in the drinking-water for 8 weeks and found clinical signs of neuropathy after 5 weeks of exposure. 2,5-Dimethylpyrrole adduct was detected in both serum and axonal cytoskeletal proteins in the exposed animals. After 2 weeks of exposure, < 1% of ε-amine groups were converted into pyrrole adducts in axonal protein. The formation of proteins of high relative molecular mass in the brain stem and spinal cord was indicative of protein cross-linking. This was associated with a loss of native neurofilament subunit proteins in the brain stem. *In vitro* incubation of axonal protein with 2,5-hexanedione also resulted in the formation of proteins of high relative molecular mass. In support of the theory that pyrrole formation is a requirement for γ-diketone neurotoxicity, DeCaprio et al. (1988) demonstrated that perdeuterio-2,5-hexanedione pyrrolylated protein at only one-third of the initial rate observed with 2,5-hexanedione, and that the deuterium analogue also caused less body weight loss than 2,5-hexanedione treatment of male Wistar rates (5 days/week, 3.5 mmol/kg per day for 17 days or 2.5 mmol/kg per day for 38 days). Hindlimb paralysis and neuropathological changes were seen only in the rats treated with 2,5-hexanedione. Pyrrole adduct concentrations were 2- to 3-fold higher in the serum and axonal cytoskeletal proteins of 2,5-hexanedione-treated rats compared with those treated with perdeuterio-2,5-hexanedione. The primary isotope effect was considered to be due to the requirement for C-H bond cleavage in pyrrole formation.

The 2,5-hexanedione analogue, 3-acetyl-2,5-hexanedione, pyrrolated protein *in vitro* at an equal rate to the potent analogue 3,4-dimethyl-2,3-hexanedione but did not form protein cross-links. Sprague-Dawley rats receiving 0.1 or 0.25 mmol 3-acetyl-2,5-hexanedione/kg per day by intraperitoneal injection and sacrificed at 20 and 7 days, respectively, did not show hindlimb paralysis or neurofilament-filled axonal swellings characteristic of γ-diketone neurotoxicity. Thus protein cross-linking appears to be a critical step in the neurotoxicity of pyrrolating agents such as 2,5-hexanedione (Genter St Clair et al., 1988). In a study of the relative effects of a range of analogues of 2,5-hexanedione, Genter et al., (1987) found a strong correlation between the rate of pyrrole formation, the rate of protein cross-linking *in vitro* and the production of neurofilament-filled axonal swellings.

Rosenberg et al. (1987b) studied male Sprague-Dawley rats given either the dl- or meso-diastereoisomers of 3,4-dimethyl-2,5-hexanedione (0.2 mmol/kg per day by intraperitoneal injection). The dl-stereoisomer produced hindlimb paralysis in one-third of the time of the meso-stereoisomer, paralleling the relative rates of *in vitro* amine pyrrolation. The more distal location of neurofilament-filled swellings after meso-3,4-dimethyl-2,5-hexanedione treatment was suggested to be due to the relatively slow rate of neurofilament cross-linking. Hyperbaric oxygen treatment made the onset of hindlimb paralysis more rapid in male Sprague-Dawley rats after daily treatment with 2,5-hexanedione (4 mmol/kg by intraperitoneal injection, 7 days/week). Rats treated with 2,5-hexanedione plus hyperbaric oxygen reached the end-point of hindlimb paralysis at 19.8 (± 1.2) days compared to 23.5 (± 0.7) days in rats treated with 2,5-hexanedione alone (p < 0.02). The results support the role of pyrrole auto-oxidation and resultant protein cross-linking in the neurotoxic process (Rosenberg et al., (1987a).

A summary of a proposed molecular mechanism linking neurofilament pyrrolylation with nerve degeneration in 2,5-hexanedione neuropathy is shown in Fig. 2.

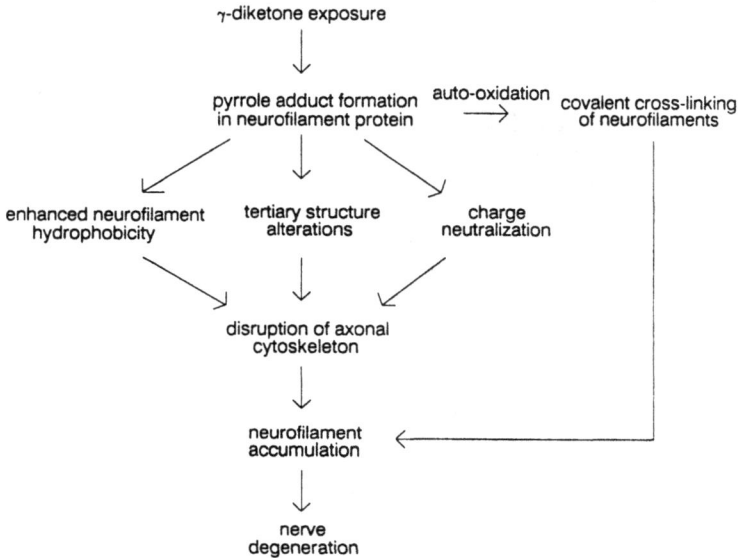

Fig. 2. Proposed scheme for nerve degeneration by 2,5-hexanedione
From: DeCaprio (1987).

Monoclonal antibodies to neurofilament proteins have been used to demonstrate protein cross-linking in the spinal cords of rats treated with 2,5-hexanedione (Lapadula et al., 1986). In male Sprague-Dawley rats given 2,5-hexanedione in drinking-water at concentrations of up to 1% (v/v) for 70 days, there was dose-dependent protein cross-linking, with decreased protein phosphorylation of neurofilament proteins and microtubulin-associated protein-2 (MAP-2) (Abou-Donia et al., 1988). The use of monoclonal antibodies to neurofilament proteins has permitted the demonstration of protein cross-linking in the spinal cords of rats treated with 2,5-hexanedione (Lapadula et al., 1986). It was also found that protein phosphorylation was decreased in association with protein cross-linking in 2,5-hexanedione-treated rats (Abou-Donia et al., 1988). It is not known if the decrease in protein phosphorylation is a primary event or a consequence of cross-linking. Exposure of three cell lines derived from human tumours or fetal mouse brain to 2,5-hexanedione *in vitro* (0.04-0.16%) resulted in reduced proliferation and an increase in cell protrusions or dendritic-like processes (Malorni et al., 1989), indicating that *in vitro* toxicity is not restricted to the neuronal system.

2,5-Hexanedione causes aggregation of intermediate filaments of the vimentin type in cultured human skin fibroblasts. Exposure to 2.8 mmol 2,5-hexanedione/litre for 1 or 2 weeks induced aggregation in 50% and 80% of the cells, respectively; a concentration of 2 mmol/litre required 2 and 3 weeks to produce corresponding effects (Durham et al., 1983). The non-neurotoxic analogues, 1,6-hexanedione and 2,4-hexanedione, had no effect on filament distribution in fibroblasts, although in the latter case cytotoxicity prevented the study of effects at concentrations equivalent to those required for 2,5-hexanedione-induced aggregation (Durham et al., 1988).

The neurotoxicity of 2,5-hexanedione was increased by co-exposure to methyl ethyl ketone (Ralston et al., 1985). Exposure to other apparently non-neurotoxic aliphatic ketones (2-pentanone, 2-heptanone, and 2-octanone) increased the neurotoxicity of the *n*-hexane metabolite 2-hexanone; 2-octanone had a greater effect than methyl ethyl ketone (Misumi & Nagano, 1985). Ladefoged et al. (1989) dosed rats with 2,5-hexanedione (0.5% in the drinking-water) for six weeks and compared the effects obtained with or without administration of 0.5% acetone or 5.0% ethanol. Nerve conduction velocity and behavioural rotarod performance were reduced after 3 weeks of dosing with 2,5-hexanedione. Acetone, but not ethanol, together with 2,5-hexanedione, had an additional significant effect on these parameters from the fourth week of dosing.

9. EFFECTS ON MAN

9.1 Single exposures

In studies on human volunteers, inhalation of 17 600 mg hexane/m^3 (5000 ppm) for 10 min resulted in vertigo and giddiness but there were no symptoms with exposure to 7040 mg/m^3 (2000 ppm) for the same duration (Patty & Yant, 1929). Occupational exposures to hexane concentrations of 3520 to 89 760 mg/m^3 (1000 to 25 500 ppm) for periods of 30-60 min caused drowsiness (Yamada, 1967).

9.2 Skin and eye irritation; sensitization

9.2.1 Skin irritation

Prolonged occlusive skin contact for 1-5 h with liquid hexane caused erythema and, after 5 h, blistering (Oettel, 1936). Application of 1.5 ml *n*-hexane (analytical grade) to 3.1 cm^2 of forearm skin for 5 min resulted in a stinging and burning sensation and transient erythema (Wahlberg, 1984a). 0.1 ml *n*-hexane rubbed gently into the forearm skin for 18 days did not produce erythema or oedema (Wahlberg, 1984b).

Operators at a soybean hexane-extraction facility had a higher incidence of dry or irritated skin than maintenance workers (65% versus 20%) (NIOSH, 1983).

9.2.2 Eye irritation

Eye irritation did not occur in volunteers exposed to hexane vapour at a level of 1760 mg/m^3 (500 ppm) for 3-5 min (Nelson et al., 1943).

9.2.3 Skin sensitization

A maximization test on 25 subjects with *n*-hexane applied undiluted for induction and as a 25% solution for challenge did not induce skin sensitization (Kligman, 1966).

9.3 Short- and long-term exposures

9.3.1 Effects on the nervous system

9.3.1.1 Peripheral neuropathy

Peripheral neuropathy has been reported in humans exposed industrially to *n*-hexane or through solvent abuse of glues or solvents containing *n*-hexane. The majority of occupational cases have occurred in small industrial concerns such as shoe manufacture in Italy and vinyl sandal production in Japan (Sobue & Yamamura, 1968; Yamamura, 1969; Inoue et al., 1970; Abbritti et al., 1976; Carapella, 1977; Palao & Lajo, 1981; Nakajima & Murayama, 1985). Workers were exposed to many volatile compounds, not only *n*-hexane, in badly ventilated rooms, sometimes for periods in excess of 8 h/day under poor hygienic conditions (Yamamura, 1969; Inoue et al., 1970, 1971; Battistini et al., 1974; Abbritti et al., 1976; Carlomagno et al., 1983).

The first signs of *n*-hexane neuropathy are symmetrical paraesthesia and weakness. The lower extremities are normally affected first. A number of other symptoms such as headache, anorexia, and dizziness may precede or coincide with the neuropathy. A "glove and stocking" sensory impairment to touch, pain, vibration, and temperature develops, with weakness and atrophy affecting proximal muscles of the extremities. On clinical examination, most patients show reduced body weight and diminished or absent reflexes. There is a marked reduction in conduction velocity in sensory and motor nerves. Electromyography (EMG) shows a neuropathic pattern including fibrillation potentials, positive sharp waves, polyphasic potentials, and reduced interference patterns. Axonal lesions of the large myelinated fibres (identical to those produced in experimental animals) with axonal swelling followed by myelin retraction at the node of Ranvier are found on nerve biopsy. There is only a slight to moderate reduction in the number of fibres, mainly of large myelinated fibres (Goto et al., 1974; Shirbae et al., 1974; Okamoto et al., 1977; Rizzuto et al., 1977, 1980; Scelsi et al., 1980; Chauplannaz et al., 1982; Lagueny et al., 1982). There are masses of 9- to 10-nm long neurofilaments in the axons. Lesions are rarely found in the small myelinated and unmyelinated fibres (Shirbae et al., 1974; Altenkirch et al., 1977; Rizzuto et al., 1977, 1980; Scelsi et al., 1980; Ruff et al., 1981; Chauplannaz et al., 1982). Muscle biopsies show signs of myofibrillar atrophy (Yamamura, 1969; Gonzalez & Downey, 1972; Shirbae et al., 1974; Altenkirch et al., 1977). Recovery is always gradual and slow and signs of residual neuropathy may persist in severe cases for 3-4 years (Yamamura, 1969; Iida & Yamamoto, 1973; Altenkirch et al., 1977; Sobue et al., 1978; Rizzuto et al., 1980; Carlomagno et al., 1983). Signs of pyramidal tract defects such as residual hyper-reflexia and spasiticity and autonomic defects have been reported in a few severe cases (Korobkin et al., 1975; Altenkirch et al., 1977; Altenkirch & Schultz, 1979; Schaumburg & Spencer, 1979). Electrophysiological evidence of central nervous system dysfunction (abnormal evoked potentials) has occasionally been reported in individual cases of peripheral neuropathy (Yoshida et al., 1974; Lagueny et al., 1982).

Neuropathy has occurred following exposure to a wide range of n-hexane levels in air from 97 to 8125 mg/m^3 (30-2500 ppm) (Oishi & Mineno, 1964; Yamada, 1964, 1967; Wada & Okamoto, 1965; Herskowitz et al., 1971; Nomiyama et al., 1973; Yoshida et al., 1974; Takeuchi et al., 1975; Paulson & Waylonis, 1976; Takahashi et al., 1977; Brugnone & Perbellini, 1980; Ono & Takeuchi, 1980; Ruff et al., 1981; Carlomagno et al., 1983). Exposure durations ranging from 2 months to 5 years may precede the onset of overt neuropathy, and a mild recurrent neuropathy with n-hexane exposure may go undetected (Wada & Okamoto, 1965; Herskowitz et al., 1971; Nomiyama et al., 1973; Takeuchi et al., 1975; Takahashi et al., 1977; Ruff et al., 1981).

In the Italian shoe industry, n-hexane (a component of the glues used) has been implicated as the cause of peripheral neuropathies (Di-Bosco & Fonzi, 1974; Abbritti et al., 1976; Cianchetti et al., 1976; Carapella, 1977; Buitatti et al., 1978; Aiello et al., 1980; Sanagi et al., 1980; Palao & Lajo, 1981; Mutti et al., 1982a,b,c).

Towfighi et al. (1976) reported the development of neuropathy in two patients who sniffed glue containing *n*-hexane. Complete clinical recovery occurred with one patient who changed to a glue not containing *n*-hexane. Sural nerve biopsies of the affected individuals indicated loss of axons. Some remaining axons had accumulation of filaments, widened nodes of Ranvier, and focal enlargements. Muscle biopsy revealed neurogenic atrophy. Three individuals in a laboratory developed neuropathy that was attributed to *n*-hexane in glue (80.4% *n*-hexane). In addition to axonal changes, the main findings were breakdown of nerve fibres and swelling and degeneration of myelin. In addition, a denervation muscle atrophy, combined with focal myopathic changes, occurred (Scelsi et al., 1981).

a) *Japanese sandal workers*

Health surveillance studies were carried out in Japan following a mass outbreak of polyneuropathy in 1967 (Sobue & Yamamura, 1968; Iida et al., 1969, Yamamura, 1969; Inoue et al., 1970, 1971; Iida & Yamamoto, 1973). Through the use of questionnaires and medical examinations, 93 cases of polyneuropathy were identified out of 1662 vinyl sandal workers who were using glues based on solvents containing more than 70% commercial grade hexane. Their work was carried out for periods of up to 14 h/day in small, badly ventilated rooms with estimated hexane air concentrations of between 1625 and 8125 mg/m^3 (500 and 2500 ppm). Air concentrations of the other volatile solvents in the glue were not described.

The workrooms were often used also as dwelling places so that continuous exposure for up to 24 h/day was possible. Clinically, the cases were classified into three groups, according to the severity of the disease:

Group I: sensory neuropathy (53 cases);
Group II: sensorimotor neuropathy (32 cases); and
Group III: motor neuropathy with amyotrophy (8 cases).

Single exposure estimations at the homes/workrooms of some of the patients indicated a positive relationship between the air concentration of hexane, the duration of the working day and the number of sandals made, and the severity of the polyneuropathy. *n*-Hexane concentrations of 1625-3250 mg/m^3 (500-1000 ppm) during an 8-h day were sufficient to cause severe peripheral neuropathy (Inoue et al., 1971).

In 89% of the cases, the onset was insidious. Initial symptoms were sensory impairment (88%), muscular weakness (14%), blurred vision (14%), coldness of extremities (13%), headache (9%), loss of body weight (9%), lassitude (3%), skin eruptions (2%), anorexia (2%), and dizziness (1%). On examination, the most common finding was a symmetrical sensorimotor disorder of the extremities. Hypoaesthesia was found in all cases and dysaesthesia was found in the early stages of the disease in 23% of patients. Other finding were muscular weakness of the limbs (43%), diminished tendon reflexes (39%), and exaggerated tendon reflexes (11%). Numbness of the face was described in five cases. Of 39 cases examined ophthalmologically, eight had abnormal findings, seven had restriction of the visual field, two had optic nerve atrophy, and one had optic neuritis. There was no correlation between the severity of neuropathy and the severity of optic effects.

Electromyography (EMG) was performed on 44 patients (11 in Group I, 25 in Group II, and 8 in Group III) (Iida et al., 1969; Yamamura, 1969). Signs of denervation, including fibrillation and positive sharp waves, were found in 70% of cases in Groups I and II and in all cases in Group III. A reduction in the number of motor units under voluntary control (reduced interference pattern) was found in 50% of cases in Group I and 70% of cases in Group III. High amplitude and polyphasic action potentials were more common in Group III than in Groups I and II. The severity of the neuropathy correlated with the type and magnitude of electromyographic abnormalities.

Motor nerve conduction velocities and evoked potentials (mixed nerve conduction velocity) were measured in the ulnar, median, peroneal, and tibial nerves in the same 44 cases. Sensory nerve conduction velocities were measured in the ulnar and median nerves. The number of cases with reduced motor nerve and sensory nerve conduction velocities correlated with the severity of the neuropathy. Reduced mixed nerve conduction velocity correlated only with the severity of neuropathy in measurements obtained from peroneal and tibial nerves.

Muscle and nerve biopsies were taken from a small number of cases. Sections of muscle showed neurogenic atrophy. Sections of nerve showed axonal and myelin lesions, and demyelination was considered to be the primary lesion (data obtained from animal studies indicate that the primary lesion in *n*-hexane neuropathy is axonal).

Polyneuropathy progressed in all severe cases (Group III) for up to 4 months after cessation of exposure. A gradual, slow recovery then ensued. Of 36 cases that were followed-up, 50%, including six severe cases (Group III), had completely or nearly completely recovered within 3-18 months. Two cases in Group III displayed residual atrophy and weakness. There were no deaths (Sobue & Yamamura, 1968; Yamamura, 1969; Inoue et al., 1970).

The clinical recovery of 90 cases was followed for approximately 5 years. Approximately 3 years after the outbreak, 51 cases had recovered completely. The remaining 39 cases were reclassified into Groups I and II (34 and 5 cases, respectively). After 5 years, 82 cases had recovered completely, while the remainder had residual sensory symptoms (Iida & Yamamoto, 1973; Sobue et al., 1978). A further study reported a significant improvement during the 5-year follow-up period in the EMG and nerve conduction velocities of some patients initially placed in Groups I and II (Iida, 1982). Patients in Group III also showed improvements in the EMG. Denervation activity and polyphasic potentials disappeared and interference patterns and high-voltage action potentials reappeared. In some patients, nerve conduction velocities were depressed for over a year after the onset of the neuropathy.

In 1981, 21 new cases of mild neuropathy were identified in the same district (Iida, 1982). Air measurements at the workplaces of the sandal makers indicated that *n*-hexane air levels were below 176 mg/m^3 (50 ppm). These cases were divided by clinical examination into 20 cases in Group I and one case in Group II. Signs of neuropathy included numbness (twelve cases), dysaesthesia (six cases), slight muscle weakness (six cases), diminished tendon reflexes (ten cases), and exaggerated tendon reflexes (three cases). Skin changes (coldness, redness, and roughness) were observed in four cases. A slight floating sensation on change of posture was reported by five patients.

EMG did not reveal any denervation in resting muscles. EMG abnormalities, more severe in the lower extremities, including reduced interference pattern, large amplitude, and polyphasic potentials, were recorded during voluntary muscle contraction in approximately 75% of cases. Significant reductions in motor or sensory nerve conduction velocities were reported in nearly half the patients.

b) *Italian shoe industry*

A study of exposure to organic solvents was carried out in an Italian shoe factory (Mutti et al., 1982a). The exposed group consisted of 95 workers (24 males, 71 females) with an age range of 16-62 years (mean, 30.9 ± 11.7 years), and the exposure duration ranged from 1 to 25 years (mean, 9.1 ± 8 years). The approximate mean air concentrations in the breathing zone, over a 2-year period, for a number of solvents were: *n*-hexane, 317 mg/m^3 (90 ppm); cyclohexane, 315 mg/m^3 (92 ppm); methyl ethyl ketone, 115 mg/m^3 (39 ppm); and ethyl acetate, 205 mg/m^3 (57 ppm). A concurrent reference group from the same factory of 52 non-exposed workers (12 males, 40 females) with an age range of 16-58 years (mean, 29.6 ± 12.3 years) and an employment duration ranging from 4 months to 29 years (mean, 10.2 months ± 9.7 years) was selected. Both exposed and reference workers underwent detailed physical examination and electrophysiological studies of the median, ulnar, and peroneal nerves. An exposure score (work time in years multiplied by an estimate of total solvent exposure) was calculated for each of the exposed workers.

Acute and chronic neurological signs and symptoms that were more frequently reported by, or found in, the exposed workers included sleepiness, dizziness, weakness, paraesthesia, and hypoaesthesia. Other neurological symptoms, such as headache, muscular cramps, neurasthenic syndrome, and sleep disturbances, were found more often in exposed workers, but the differences in incidence between the exposed and reference group were not statistically significant. Some parameters of electrophysiological measurements indicated subclinical neuropathy among exposed workers. The mean motor nerve conduction velocity was significantly reduced in the median and peroneal nerves but not in the ulnar nerve. The amplitude of the motor action potential (MAP) was significantly reduced in all nerves and its duration was increased in the ulnar nerve. There were no significant effects on the distal latency. A significantly higher number of abnormal action potentials was observed in the median and peroneal nerves of exposed workers. There was a correlation between the reduction in motor conduction velocity and the exposure score, but not with age of the individual. Comparison of the electrophysiological parameters between two exposed sub-groups and the reference group indicated an exposure-related trend for reduced motor conduction velocity in the median and peroneal nerves, and an increased motor action potential amplitude duration.

When the 95 exposed workers were divided into two sub-groups based on *n*-hexane exposure, 65 workers having low exposure (243 mg/m^3, 69 ppm) and 30 having high exposure (475 mg/m^3, 135 ppm), there was an exposure-related trend in the reduction of median nerve motor conduction velocity and increase in the duration of the ulnar nerve motor action potential (Mutti et al., 1982b).

In a follow-up study, electrophysiological measurements including somatosensory evoked potentials (SEPs) were recorded from a group of 15 women shoe factory workers aged 19-53 years (mean age, 26.6 ± 11.4 years) with an exposure duration to solvents of 2-8 years (mean, 4.5 ± 2.3 years) (Mutti et al., 1982c). The mean air concentrations for various solvents in the breathing zone of the workers were: *n*-hexane, 690 mg/m^3 (196 ppm); cyclohexane, 585 mg/m^3 (170 ppm); methyl ethyl ketone, 177 mg/m^3 (60 ppm); and ethyl acetate, 360 mg/m^3 (100 ppm). However, total solvent levels occasionally exceeded 5000-7000 mg/m^3 when the ventilation system failed. The study started 3 months after hygiene improvements successfully controlled air levels of solvents. A control group of 15 age- and health-matched women was used.

Electrophysiological measurements in peripheral nerves showed significant reductions in maximal motor and distal sensory nerve conduction velocities in the median and ulnar nerves and reduced maximal motor nerve conduction velocity in the peroneal nerve. The latency of the sensory peak action potential was significantly increased in the median and ulnar nerves. The amplitude of all peripheral nerve action potentials was slightly reduced but this was not statistically significant.

There were changes in the somatosensory evoked potentials (SEPs) of exposed workers with significant increases in the latency of some early component peaks. The amplitude of some of the early peaks was also increased, but the amplitude of the later peaks was significantly reduced. Comparison of SEPs from exposed and non-exposed workers showed that later components in exposed workers were flatter.

An electrophysiological study was carried out on 25 workers (13 women, 12 men), placed into two groups according to job specification, out of 31 workers at an Italian shoe factory (Aiello et al., 1980). Group A contained 11 subjects (seven women and four men), aged 21-50 years with 0.3 to 20 years of exposure, who worked in direct contact with solvents. Group B contained 14 subjects (six women and eight men), aged 20-49 years and exposed for 0.25-20 years, who had no direct contact with solvents but were exposed by inhalation. Peak values for air concentrations of various solvents in the factory were: n-hexane, 70 mg/m^3 (20 ppm); ethyl acetate, 1.8 mg/m^3 (0.5 ppm); cyclohexane, 620 mg/m^3 (40 ppm); and trichloroethylene, 2.7 mg/m^3 (0.5 ppm).

Motor nerve conduction velocity was measured in the median and peroneal nerves, and sensory nerve conduction velocity in the median and ulnar nerves. The distal latency and amplitude of action potentials were measured in motor and in sensory fibres.

Statistically significant electrophysiological changes were found in seven workers from Group A. An increased distal latency in sensory or motor fibres was found in six of these workers and reduced motor nerve conduction velocity in the peroneal nerve in one worker. In three workers from Group B, there was a significant increase in the distal latency in sensory nerves of the upper limb. In one of these, there was reduced motor nerve conduction velocity. EMG abnormalities were detected in two workers, one from each group. Seven out of 14 workers exposed for more than 5 years exhibited one or more electrophysiological abnormalities. In three out of eight workers exposed for between 1 and 5 years, there were abnormal findings. There were no abnormalities in the three workers with less than one year's exposure.

c) *Taiwan press proofing workers*

In a cross-sectional survey among Taiwanese press proofers, using solvents containing *n*-hexane to clean machinery, workers from 16 factories who had been employed in the industry for more than 2 months underwent detailed neurological examination (Wang et al., 1986). A total of 59 workers (57 males, and 2 females) with a mean age of 25.8 (± 10.2) years and a mean employment duration of 5.8 years (range, 2 months to 25 years) was examined. Nerve conduction velocity studies were undertaken in 54 workers, and a diagnosis of peripheral neuropathy was made on the basis of objective clinical signs compatible with peripheral neuropathy and at least two abnormally slow conduction velocities (45 m/sec in the upper extremities and 40 m/sec in the lower extremities). Mean nerve conduction velocities for the exposed group were compared with a control group of 150 individuals (50 in each of the age ranges 10-35, 36-50, and 51-80 years). The sex ratio of the control group was not provided and exposed and control groups were not matched for age.

n-Hexane was present in samples of the commercial solvents used to clean the machines from all the factories at concentrations of between 3 and 65%. Post-event measurements of *n*-hexane air concentrations (14 factories) varied from 0 to 669 mg/m^3 (190 ppm). Prior to the discovery of neuropathy, standards of hygiene were described as poor. Groups of 3-9 workers cleaned press proof machines in small poorly ventilated rooms for more than 8 h/day.

Fifteen cases of overt peripheral neuropathy were diagnosed among exposed workers (14 males, and 1 female; employment range, 6 months to 5 years; median, 1.5 years). Sural nerve biopsies from three cases were consistent with *n*-hexane peripheral neuropathy. The reported *n*-hexane air concentrations for two factories where eight of these people worked were 669 mg/m^3 (190 ppm) (six cases) and

74 mg/m^3 (21 ppm) (two cases). No exposure data were available for the remaining seven cases employed in one factory. Twelve of the 15 cases regularly slept in the factory and were exposed to *n*-hexane for daily periods in excess of 8 h.

Exposure to *n*-hexane air concentrations of less than 352 mg/m^3 (100 ppm) was not associated with clinical peripheral neuropathy. There were significant reductions in the median, ulnar, and peroneal nerve mean motor nerve conduction velocities in the *n*-hexane-exposed workers without diagnosed peripheral neuropathy, compared with the control group, but an exposure-related trend was not found.

In a subsequent neurological investigation of workers at these factories, there was evidence of central nervous system malfunction, indicated by somatosensory and visual evoked responses, in individuals with peripheral neuropathy and also in other workers (Chang, 1985). Twenty-two of the polyneuropathy cases, five subclinical cases and seven unaffected workers were investigated. The absolute and interpeak latencies of patterned visual evoked potential in affected cases were longer than in normal controls, and the evoked potential interpeak amplitude was decreased in individuals with polyneuropathy (Chang, 1987). Effects on the brainstem auditory evoked response (BAER) were also reported (Chang, 1985). Wave I latency between factory workers and normal controls did not differ, but prolongation of the wave I-V interpeak latencies was noted in workers and corresponded to the severity of polyneuropathy. Five factory workers exposed to *n*-hexane for 5-30 months had a reduction in nerve conduction velocity that was correlated with clinical signs (Huang & Chu, 1989). Neurological symptoms consisted of muscle cramp and weakness, distal numbness, and, in one case, blurred vision and tinnitus. The tibial-central conduction in the somatosensory evoked potentials was delayed and the central conduction time of the BAER was also prolonged, indicating primary defects in the spinal cord and brainstem.

d) *Tungsten carbide milling*

The effect of exposure to *n*-hexane was investigated in a factory producing tungsten carbide alloys where powders of tungsten carbide and other metals and carbides were mixed with *n*-hexane or acetone by ball mills (Sanagi et al., 1980). Fourteen workers (concurrently exposed), aged less than 50 with exposure durations of 1-12 years (mean, 6.2 years), who were engaged in the ball milling and drying of tungsten carbide alloys were studied. A further group (previously exposed) of five workers, aged less than 50 with exposure durations of 1-16 years (mean, 5.2 years), who had worked in ball milling in the past were also investigated. Workers exhibiting any evidence of neurological disorders were excluded from this study. A concurrent control group of 14 workers not exposed to *n*-hexane was selected from the sintering workshop. The mean 8-h time-weighted average concentration of *n*-hexane over a 2-year period was 204 mg/m^3 (58 ppm). The average concentrations for acetone were in the range 52-164 mg per m^3 (22-69 ppm). The medical history of each worker was assessed by interview and questionnaire. Neurological status was determined by detailed clinical examination and electrophysiological studies.

Headaches, hyperaesthesia in the limbs, and muscle weakness tended to be reported more often by workers in the exposed group. Neurological examination did not reveal any abnormalities of cranial nerves, the pyramidal tract, or peripheral motor nerves. Paraesthesia was noted in three exposed subjects and one control subject. There was a slightly higher prevalence of diminished bicipital and patellar tendon reflexes in the exposed group. There were significant effects on muscle strength (jump test on one foot) and vibration sensation (tuning fork) when mean values for the exposed groups were compared with the control group. Electrophysiological measurements showed no signs of neuropathy in any worker, but in the concurrently exposed group mean maximal motor conduction velocities in the posterior tibial nerve were significantly reduced compared with those of the control group. In addition, the mean distal latency in the posterior tibial nerve was significantly increased in both the concurrently and previously exposed groups.

e) *Extraction facilities*

Two workers at a hexane extraction facility reported transient paraesthesia following excessive acute exposure to hexane. The predominant complaint at the facility was of temporary episodes of light-headedness and dizziness. The maximum time-weighted average (8 h) hexane concentration at this site was 92 mg/m^3 (26 ppm) (NIOSH, 1981a). The most frequently reported symptoms in workers associated with a soybean extraction facility were dizziness, giddiness, and light-headedness (each reported by 74% of participants). Headache and weakness were also reported by 56 and 52%, respectively, of cases. Operators had a higher incidence of sleepiness (41%) than did maintenance workers (0%). Exposure concentrations in personal breathing zones ranged from 15.5 to 46.5 mg/m^3 (4.4-13.2 ppm), but leaks from some process equipment may have led to higher levels of acute exposure (NIOSH, 1983).

f) *Maizlish study*

Workers with long-term exposure to mixtures of organic solvents have been reported to experience mild, clinically detectable, sensory or sensorimotor polyneuropathies (Husman & Karli, 1980). In a study by Maizlish et al. (1987), there was no association between impaired neurological function and solvent concentration in mixed exposure to solvents (isopropanol, naphtha, hexane) in workers occupationally exposed for an average of 6 years. Of 240 workers exposed to mixtures of these solvents, with hexane at breathing-zone concentrations of 3.5-137 mg/m^3 (1-39 ppm), 16% had presumed, but not clinically significant, signs of peripheral neuropathy (diminished pain response, vibratory sensation, and ankle reflex). The signs were not related to solvent exposure concentration. Overall, the relative risk (RR = 1.4) of the presumed signs of peripheral neuropathy was not statistically significant.

9.3.1.2 *Effects on vision and optic nerves*

Blurred vision has been reported in some cases of peripheral neuropathy attributed to *n*-hexane exposure (Wada & Okamoto, 1965; Sobue & Yamamura, 1968; Yamamura, 1969). No effects on visual acuity or on the optic fundus have been reported in case histories of peripheral neuropathy where information on ophthalmic examinations was provided (Wada et al., 1965; Yamamura, 1969; Shirbae et al., 1974).

Constriction of the visual field, optic neuritis, and optic atrophy were reported in one study on Japanese vinyl sandal makers with peripheral neuropathy (Rizzuto et al., 1980).

In a study of the ocular effects of n-hexane, 15 workers (11 males, 4 females) making adhesive bandages or extracting vegetable oils, aged 30-65 (mean age, 46 years) with exposure durations of 5-21 years (mean exposure, 12 years), were examined ophthalmologically and given colour discrimination tests and fluorescein angiography (Raitta et al., 1978). Eight workers were from adhesive bandage factories where peak n-hexane air concentrations were 1489, 2126, and 3992 mg/m^3 (423, 604, and 1134 ppm) around a glue-spreading machine, 1866 and 4506 mg/m^3 (530 and 1280 ppm) at an opened mixing machine, and 11 440 mg/m^3 (3250 ppm) at floor level near a tape machine. Air levels of n-hexane in the breathing zone of workers were lower than these values and n-hexane air levels in the factories were generally below 1760 mg/m^3 (500 ppm). Seven individuals worked in the extraction of vegetable oils at a factory where the n-hexane air concentrations in the processing room were between 35 and 176 mg/m^3 (10 and 50 ppm), although air levels as high as 7040-10 560 mg/m^3 (2000-3000 ppm) could be reached when processing was interrupted. There was no control group.

In three individuals (two of whom had pre-existing defects) there were disturbances in visual acuity or field of vision. Colour vision defects, mainly blue-yellow, were found in 12 workers. There were no cases of optic atrophy. In nine workers the maculae showed slight pigment dystrophy, in three there were yellowish dots, and in one the foveal reflex was absent. Fluorescein angiography showed patchy choroidal underfilling, capillary widening of the perifoveal arcade, and loss of retinal pigment around the macula. Colour discrimination defects and maculopathy appeared to be related.

In a subsequent study, visual evoked potentials and electroretinograms (ERGs) were recorded in the same 15 workers and compared with control measurements obtained from 10 healthy subjects aged 21-57 (mean age, 34.9 years) who were not occupationally exposed to solvents (Seppalainen et al., 1979). There were significant reductions in peak-to-peak amplitudes for a number of visual evoked potential components, possibly due to conduction block in intracerebral axons. The latency of several components was significantly increased. This was attributed to partial axonal degeneration in the visual pathways. A significant decrease in the amplitude of the electroretinogram (ERG) was reported, with a reduced latency in the "b" wave. The effects on the ERG in the exposed workers could not be correlated directly with the effects on retinal pigments and colour discrimination reported by Raitta et al. (1978). Seppalainen & Raitta (1981) found electroneuromyographic signs of peripheral neuropathy, including reduced nerve conduction velocity and/or fibrillation or long duration motor unit potentials, in 11 of the 15 workers. Symptoms included "drunkenness" (8), headache (7), tiredness (5), and paraesthesia in the limbs (5). All workers with paraesthesia had at least one electrophysiological sign of neuropathy. Abnormal EEG findings (slow wave abnormalities) were found in 9 of the workers.

Signs of maculopathy and colour discrimination defects were noted in 10 out of the 11 workers with abnormal electrophysiological signs or peripheral neuropathy. Colour discrimination defects were present in 8 of the 9 workers with EEG abnormalities. There were altered EMG and EEG traces in 6 of the 12 workers with colour discrimination defects. The authors suggested that there was a correlation between maculopathy and peripheral neuropathy.

Abnormal visual evoked potentials were reported in a study of glue sniffers exposed to *n*-hexane (Cooper et al., 1985). Abnormal electro-physiological signs persisted in two individuals who were retested 6 months after they had stopped inhaling solvents. However, these individuals had been exposed to a wide range of organic solvents and exposure information was inadequate.

In somatosensory evoked potentials, both the absolute latencies and central conduction time were prolonged in affected workers (Chang, 1987). In a study of 25 patients, 5 subclinical cases, and 45 apparently healthy workers, Chang & Yip (1987) reported various electrophysiological abnormalities that reflected, in polyneuropathy patients, pathological changes of primary giant axonal degeneration with secondary myelinopathy. This was based on the observation of a marked fall in nerve conduction velocities, profound amplitude reduction of muscle action potentials and sensory action potentials and, prolongation of latencies. Early electroneurographic changes in the apparently healthy individuals exposed to n-hexane were reduction in the nerve conduction velocities, prolongation of motor distal latency, and attenuation of sensory action potential amplitude.

9.3.2 *Effects on the kidney*

An investigation of kidney function was conducted on a group of 64 workers (age and sex not reported) exposed for 1-24 years to hydrocarbon mixtures at a shoe factory and an undefined control group of 80 subjects (Nakajima & Murayama, 1985). Mean air concentrations for solvents in the factory over a period of one year were: n-hexane, 250 mg/m^3 (71 ppm); cyclohexane, 203 mg/m^3 (59 ppm); methyl ethyl ketone, 44 mg/m^3 (15 ppm); and ethyl acetate, 180 mg/m^3 (50 ppm). No effects on mean total urinary protein, albumin, β-glucuronidase, or muramidase levels were reported.

A study of kidney function was also undertaken on a group of 182 Italian shoe workers selected from 185 workers employed at four factories (59 males, 123 females; mean age, 39.4 years; mean exposure duration, 10.2 years) (Mutti et al., 1981; Franchini et al., 1983). Breathing-zone concentrations were estimated for a number of solvents (hexane, ethyl acetate, cyclohexane, methyl ethyl ketone, and acetone), and concentrations of hexane (n-hexane and 2- and 3-methylpentane) were reported to be significantly higher than 100 ppm (352 mg n-hexane per m^3) on a number of occasions. Eighty healthy subjects (30 males, 50 females; mean age, 37.9 years) without a history of renal disease or exposure to organic solvents were used as a control group. A further control group of 30 unexposed workers (10 males, 20 females; mean age, 41.6 years) was randomly selected from 124 workers who had left the factories during the previous 5 years (mean exposure duration, 8.8 years).

Spot samples of urine were analysed for total protein, albumin, and creatinine levels and for β-glucuronidase activity. Urinary lysozyme activity was estimated in a few workers. Blood samples were analysed for creatinine levels. The mean total urinary protein level was significantly higher in the exposed workers than in either control or historically exposed workers. Seven workers (4 males, 3 females) had abnormally high levels (greater than two standard deviations of the mean control value). Four of these workers also had abnormally high urinary lysozyme activity, and two had increased β-glucuronidase activity. There were no effects on urinary albumin or serum creatinine levels.

9.3.3 Effects on other organs

Health surveillance studies were carried out in Japan following a mass outbreak of polyneuropathy in 1967 (Sobue & Yamamura, 1968, Iida et al., 1969, Yamamura, 1969; Inoue et al., 1970, 1971; Iida & Yamamoto, 1973).

No effects on the respiratory system, kidney, liver, or haematopoietic organs were reported.

Laboratory examinations were inconsistent. Urinalysis showed positive urobilinogen in 15 cases and raised coproporphyrin levels in four cases. The cephalin cholesterol flocculation test was positive in 9 cases and a slight to moderately raised serum lactate dehydrogenase level was found in 17 cases. Depressed cholinesterase levels were reported in 26 out of 42 cases examined. There was no correlation between the depressed cholinesterase levels and severity of neuropathy. The cerebrospinal fluid was examined in 7 cases and was normal, with no significant effect on pressure or protein levels. Plethysmography was performed in 11 cases and weak vasomotor responses were found in two cases.

10. EVALUATION OF HUMAN HEALTH RISKS AND EFFECTS ON THE ENVIRONMENT

10.1 Animal studies

10.1.1 Short- and long-term exposure

n-Hexane is of low acute toxicity, LD_{50} values in the range 15-30 g/kg and an LC_{50} (1 h) of 271 040 mg per m^3 having been reported.

In essentially continuous inhalation studies in rats, deaths occurred following n-hexane exposure to 3520 mg per m^3 (1000 ppm) for up to 11 weeks, and reduced body weight gain after 3 weeks of exposure to 1760 mg/m^3 (500 ppm). In studies involving daily 12-h exposures to n-hexane, deaths were recorded at 10 560 mg/m^3 (3000 ppm) after 15 weeks and slightly reduced body weight gain at 740 mg per m^3 (200 ppm) after 24 weeks. No effects on body weight were noted in rats exposed to 443 mg/m^3 (126 ppm) virtually continuously for 34 weeks.

Testicular toxicity and peripheral and central neurotoxicity appear to be the principal non-lethal effects of repeated n-hexane exposure in rats. Severe testicular lesions have resulted from inhalation exposure to n-hexane and oral exposure to 2,5-hexanedione. Effects have been attributed to disruption of the cytoskeleton of Sertoli cells. There are secondary effects on post-spermatogonial germ cells, which disappear from affected tubules. Testicular effects were reversible after a single exposure for 24 h to 17 600 mg/m^3 (5000 ppm) but irreversible after a 2-weeks exposure to the same concentration for 16 h/day, 6 days/week. 2,5-Hexanedione at 1% in drinking water produced reversible testicular lesions after 2 to 3 weeks of dosing and irreversible effects (within 17 weeks) after 5 weeks of dosing.

Clinically, neurotoxicity is characterized by hindlimb weakness, which can progress to paralysis and eventually to quadriplegia. Clinical signs have been seen after 10 weeks of discontinuous exposure to 10 560 mg/m^3 (3000 ppm) (12 h/day, 7 days/week) and after 6-10 weeks of continuous exposure to 1408 to 2112 mg/m^3 (400 to 600 ppm).

Lesions (axonal swellings) in hindlimb nerves, brain, and spinal cord have been observed prior to the appearance of hindlimb weakness. More severe effects (axonal degeneration and loss) were noted, particularly in the longest nerves with the largest diameter, after 6 months of exposure to 1760 mg/m^3 (500 ppm). Overall, no-observed-adverse-effect levels for *n*-hexane-induced neurotoxicity in rats are difficult to establish because of the range of vapour concentrations and exposure regimes tested, and the variety of effects investigated. In essentially continuous 6-month inhalation studies, nerve lesions were seen at *n*-hexane concentrations of 1760 mg per m^3 (500 ppm) or more, but no clinical or pathological effects were noted at 440 mg/m^3 (125 ppm). Discontinuous exposure of rats to 3168 mg/m^3 (900 ppm) for 72 weeks did not cause any apparent nerve lesions, but there was some preliminary evidence for an effect on grip strength.

Resolution (partial or complete) of clinical signs of toxicity, reduced grip strength, and electrophysiological effects can occur following cessation of exposure. Only limited recovery of amplitude of the fifth component of the brainstem auditory-evoked response component (believed to reflect central nervous system activity) and tail nerve action potential was recorded 15 to 22 weeks after the end of repeated exposure to 3520 mg/m^3 (1000 ppm) for 11 weeks. Resolution of pathological lesions has not been systematically investigated following inhalation exposure, but remyelination and limited axonal regeneration have been observed following cessation of exposure to 1408 to 2112 mg/m^3 (400 to 600 ppm).

Inhalation of 1760 mg/m^3 (500 ppm) discontinuously for 7 weeks can cause minor damage to the lungs of rats. In rabbits, severe respiratory tract lesions were seen following exposure to 10 560 mg/m^3 (3000 ppm), 8 h/day for 8 days, and papillary proliferations of non-ciliated bronchiolar cells were noted after 24 weeks of exposure.

Effects on the kidney and liver have been reported in a few inhalation studies on rats but only at higher exposure levels. Most lesions and other effects were considered to be of minor toxicological significance and/or were not reproducible in repeated studies. However, severe liver lesions have been noted in rats following repeated intraperitoneal administration of *n*-hexane.

Combined exposure studies have shown that the neurotoxic effects of *n*-hexane vapour can be enhanced in hens by methyl isobutyl ketone (MIBK) and in rats by both methyl ethyl ketone and lead acetate, but decreased by toluene. Pulmonary lesions in rats have also been reported to be enhanced by co-exposure to methyl ethyl ketone.

There have been few studies on the effects of oral or dermal exposure to *n*-hexane. Daily oral administration of 500 mg/kg per day for 4 weeks resulted in reduced tail nerve conduction velocity in rats.

10.1.2 Genotoxicity

Only limited mutagenicity testing has been conducted. Chromosomal damage (polyploidy in one study, structural aberrations in a second study) was reported in *in vitro* assays in which a Chinese hamster cell line was exposed to undiluted liquid *n*-hexane in the absence of a metabolizing fraction. No significant increase in point mutation rate occurred in cultured mammalian cells or bacteria following exposure to *n*-hexane. DNA damage, as measured in differential bacterial toxicity assays, was not increased by exposure to *n*-hexane. Similarly, no increase in unscheduled DNA synthesis was noted in human lymphocytes *in vitro*. Although *n*-hexane has given negative results in assays for point mutations there is some evidence that it can produce chromosomal aberrations *in vitro*. Chromosomal damage (chromatid breaks) in rat bone marrow cells was reported in an *in vivo* study.

10.1.3 Carcinogenicity

The carcinogenic potential of *n*-hexane has not been adequately studied. In a limited study, dermally applied *n*-hexane did not appear to enhance the formation of skin tumours in mice following exposure to a tumour initiator (7,12-dimethylbenzanthracene) or co-exposure with a promoting agent (croton oil).

4

10.1.4 Reproductive effects

The reproductive toxicity of *n*-hexane has not been adequately investigated. There is no substantial evidence of embryotoxicity or teratogenicity in rats following inhalation or in mice after oral dosing. Slight increases in the incidence of some anomalies were noted in rats exposed to 10 560 mg/m^3 (3000 ppm), but inadequacies in the conduct of the study (e.g., the concentration tested was probably not high enough) limit the conclusions that can be reached. Signs of fetotoxicity (reduced pup weight) were noted in mice, but only at doses that resulted in significant maternal mortality. A transient delay in postnatal development was reported in one study in the pups of rats exposed to 10 560 mg/m^3 (3000 ppm). Although no signs of neuropathy were reported in these animals, it is not possible to assess from this study whether *in utero* exposure could induce neuropathy, as the animals were only exposed to *n*-hexane during a small part of the gestation period. Other reports have claimed that *in utero* exposure to *n*-hexane retards cerebellar histogenesis and neuronal maturation and induces electrophysiological abnormalities of the central nervous system in neonatal rats. However, this work has not been reported in sufficient detail for a full assessment to be made.

There is evidence that *n*-hexane causes irreversible sterility in the rat. No effects on male fertility were reported in a limited dominant lethal study on the mouse. No investigations of fertility in female animals or multi-generation studies have been reported.

10.2 Human studies

10.2.1 Effects on the nervous system

Many studies have linked occupational *n*-hexane exposure to the incidence of peripheral neuropathy in humans. However, few of these studies reported air concentrations, those reported may be inaccurate, and it is often not clear whether these concentrations are of hexane or *n*-hexane. In addition, industrial exposure to *n*-hexane usually occurs during the use of solvent-based products, so workers are exposed to a mixture of volatile compounds (e.g., ethyl acetate, methyl ethyl ketone, toluene, acet-one, and other aliphatic hydrocarbons). Air concentrations for the other solvents present have rarely been documen-ted. Only those studies that present some air concen-tration data have been included in this review.

The results of peripheral nerve electrophysiology may vary considerably depending on the type of technique used, the ambient temperature at which measurements are taken, the segment of the nerve studied, and the age of the individual. Thus, the assessment of studies that rely on peripheral nerve electrophysiology is difficult in the absence of information on these factors.

Studies on 93 cases of neuropathy characterized the clinical features of *n*-hexane neuropathy and showed that electrophysiological measurements correlated well with the severity of the condition. An association between increas-ing severity of the disease and increasing exposure was found. However, from the limited details of exposure reported, it was not possible to establish any definite relationship.

Mild subclinical signs of neuropathy were found in shoe workers exposed to 70 mg/m^3 (20 ppm). The degree of electrophysiological abnormalities increased with duration of exposure. However, no cases of overt neuropathy oc-curred, even in workers with an exposure duration longer than 5 years.

Subjective and electrophysiological signs of subclini-cal peripheral neuropathy were found in a group of workers exposed to approximately 317 mg/m^3 (90 ppm). However, these effects cannot be wholly ascribed to exposure to this level of *n*-hexane, since previous exposure to sol-vents was probably underestimated and worker self-selection may have introduced bias. In addition, there may have been co-exposure to methyl ethyl ketone, which has been demonstrated to enhance the neurotoxic effects of *n*-hexane.

Exposure to a solvent mixture containing an *n*-hexane level of approximately 690 mg/m^3 (196 ppm) resulted in reduced nerve conduction velocity along peripheral nerves, which persisted after exposure had been significantly reduced. In addition, an effect of *n*-hexane on the central nervous system has been suggested to be the cause of some of the somatosensory evoked potential changes noted.

Subjective and electrophysiological signs of mild subclinical neuropathy occurred in a small group of workers exposed to mean *n*-hexane concentrations in air of 208 mg/m³ (59 ppm). Clinical overt neuropathy was not detected. In this study exposure to other solvents was limited and the nerve conduction studies were performed under defined conditions. However, the small number of subjects studied, lack of historical exposure data, and the poor matching of the exposed and control groups limit the value of the conclusions reached. Nevertheless, the results are in general agreement with the data obtained in the earlier studies reported above. Exposure to 669 mg/m³ (190 ppm) for periods in excess of 8 h/day was associated with the onset of clinically overt peripheral neuropathy. Partial recovery of nerve function can occur slowly over several years. Exposure to less than 352 mg/m³ (100 ppm) did not result in neuropathy but showed electrophysiological evidence of subclinical effects.

Colour discrimination defects and signs of maculopathy have been described in a small number of workers occupationally exposed to a wide range of *n*-hexane levels in air. Visual-evoked potential and electroretinogram measurements of these individuals showed abnormalities compared with a control group of non-exposed workers. Abnormal visual-evoked potential traces have also been reported in some glue sniffers exposed to *n*-hexane. It has been suggested that axonal degeneration may occur in the visual pathway and that *n*-hexane may induce a central nerve conduction block. There is also some evidence that signs of maculopathy may be correlated with electrophysiological signs of peripheral neuropathy. Abnormal EEG traces were also found in some of the individuals studied.

10.2.2 Other effects

No studies have been reported on fertility or possible testicular effects in males. Very little information is available on the acute toxicity of *n*-hexane to humans. Most studies have involved exposure to solvent mixtures.

The available data suggest that *n*-hexane is of low acute toxicity.

Very few studies of skin or eye irritancy involving volunteers have been published. *n*-Hexane is a mild irritant causing transient erythema when in contact with human skin for short periods. More severe effects (erythema and blistering) were documented after occlusive skin contact for 5 h to commercial grade hexane. Insufficient data are available to assess whether the liquid can cause eye irritation in human beings. No signs of eye irritation were noted in a study in which volunteers were exposed to a hexane vapour concentration of 1760 mg/m^3 (500 ppm) for 3-5 min. There have been no reports of skin sensitization in exposed workers and no skin sensitization was noted in a maximization test with *n*-hexane.

10.3 Environmental effects

n-Hexane has low solubility in water and is highly volatile. Exposure of aquatic organisms is, therefore, likely to be low and transient except for uncontrolled discharges into surface waters. Data on the toxicity of *n*-hexane to aquatic organisms are few, variable, conducted under inappropriate conditions and inadequate to make an assessment of this environmental risk.

11. RECOMMENDATIONS

11.1 Human health protection

At the levels of n-hexane to which the general population is exposed, there is unlikely to be any hazard. In the occupational health context, atmospheric levels should be kept below the recommended occupational exposure limits by suitably designed work processes and engineering controls including ventilation. Suitable protective clothing and respiratory protection should be readily available for use in enclosed spaces, in emergencies, and for certain maintenance operations. The use of a supplied-air respirator or a self-contained breathing apparatus in continuous flow mode for n-hexane concentrations up to 8800 mg/m³ (2500 ppm) is recommended. It should be fitted with a full facepiece for concentrations between 8800 mg/m³ (2500 ppm) and 17 600 mg/m³ (5000 ppm). Although protective gloves may resist penetration by n-hexane, mixtures of n-hexane with other solvents, such as methyl ethyl ketone, may permit the n-hexane to penetrate gloves and other protective clothing. This factor should be considered when using n-hexane mixtures.

11.2 Environmental protection

n-Hexane is unlikely to present a hazard to the environment, except in the case of major spills or discharges where there could be transient local effects.

12. FURTHER RESEARCH

a) A study of indices of testicular function should be made in an occupationally exposed group(s) to establish whether any or all of the effects reported to occur in the testes of animals are also manifested in man.

b) The genotoxic effects of *n*-hexane should be further investigated *in vivo* in order to supplement the limited *in vitro* information on genotoxicity.

c) A repeat dose study is required to establish the toxicity of *n*-hexane given by the oral route. This is needed to provide a NOEL in order to establish an ADI.

d) The mechanism of neurotoxicity at the molecular level is not clear. Understanding the mechanism will contribute directly to the validity of risk assessment. *In vivo* and *in vitro* studies are required to investigate further and clarify these mechanisms.

e) Available teratogenicity studies are inadequate for an evaluation of risk. Studies should be undertaken to provide usable data.

f) Dose-response relationships concerning neurotoxic effects of *n*-hexane in humans are unclear because of incomplete or unreliable exposure data. Moreover, although peripheral neurotoxicity by *n*-hexane has been amply demonstrated, effects on the central nervous system have been explored only to a limited extent. Further epidemiological investigations such as prospective follow-up studies should be undertaken in order to overcome the shortcomings of previous investigations.

REFERENCES

ABBRITTI, G., SIRACUSA, A., CIANCHETTI, C., COLI, C.A., CURRADI, F., PERTICONI, G.F., & DE ROSA, F. (1976) Shoe makers' polyneuropathy in Italy: the aetiological problem. Br. J. ind. Med., 33: 92-99.

ABDEL-RAHMAN, M.S., HETLAND, L.B., & COURI, D. (1976) Toxicity and metabolism of methyl n-butyl ketone. Am. Ind. Hyg. Assoc. J., 37: 95-102.

ABE, K., MISUMI, J., KAWAKAMI, M., & NOMURA, S. (1980) Effects of n-hexane, methyl n-butyl ketone, and 2,5-hexanedione on the excitability of sweat glands in rats to mecholyl. Jpn. J. ind. Health, 22: 380-381.

ABOU-DONIA, M.B., LAPADULA, D.M., CAMPBELL, G., & TIMMONS, P.R. (1985a) The synergism of n-hexane-induced neurotoxicity by methyl isobutyl ketone following subchronic (90 days) inhalation in hens: Induction of hepatic microsomal cytochrome P-450. Toxicol. appl. Pharmacol., 81: 1-16.

ABOU-DONIA, M.B., MAKKAWY, H.M., & CAMPBELL, G.M. (1985b) Pattern of neurotoxicity of n-hexane, methyl n-butyl ketone, 2,5-hexanediol, and 2,5-hexanedione alone and in combination with 0-ethyl 0-4-nitrophenyl phenylphosphonothioate in hens. J. Toxicol. environ. Health, 16: 85-100.

ABOU-DONIA, M.B., LAPADULA, D.M., & SUWITA, E. (1988) Cytoskeletal proteins as targets for organophosphorus compound and aliphatic hexacarbon-induced neurotoxicity. Toxicology, 49: 469-477.

ACGIH (1986) Documentation of the threshold limit values, 5th ed., Cincinnati, Ohio, American Conference of Governmental Industrial Hygienists.

AHONEN, I. & SCHIMBERG, R.W. (1988) 2,5-hexanedione excretion after occupational exposure to n-hexane. Br. J. ind. Med., 45: 133-136.

AIELLO, I., ROSATI, G., SERRA, G., & MANCA, M. (1980) Subclinical neuropathic disorders and precautionary measures in the shoe industry. An electrophysiological investigation. Acta neurol. (Napoli), 35: 285-292.

ALTENKIRCH, H. & SCHULTZ, H. (1979) [Glue sniffing and neuropathy. Neurological findings and social data from 40 cases.] Nervenarzt, 50: 21-27 (in German).

ALTENKIRCH, H., MAGER, J., STOLTENBURG, G., & HELMBRECHT, J. (1977) Toxic polyneuropathies after sniffing a glue thinner. J. Neurol., 214: 137-152.

ALTENKIRCH, H., STOLTENBURG-DIDINGER, G., & WAGNER, H.M. (1978) Experimental studies on hydrocarbon neuropathies induced by methyl ethyl ketone (MEK). J. Neurol., 219: 159-170.

ALTENKIRCH, H., STOLTENBURG-DIDINGER, G., & WAGNER, H.M. (1979) Experimental data on the neurotoxicity of methyl ethyl ketone (MEK). Experientia (Basel), 35: 503-504.

ALTENKIRCH, H., WAGNER, H.M., STOLTENBURG, G., & SPENCER, P.S. (1982) Nervous system responses of rats to subchronic inhalation of n-hexane and n-hexane plus methyl ethyl ketone mixtures. J. neurol. Sci., 57: 209-219.

ANDERSON, R.J. & DUNHAM, C.B. (1984) Electrophysiologic deficits in peripheral nerve as a discriminator of early hexacarbon neurotoxicity. J. Toxicol. environ. Health, 13: 835-843.

ANGELO, M.J. (1977) The pharmacokinetics of the neurotoxin 2,5-hexanedione: distribution, elimination and model simulations, Newark, University of Delaware (Ph.D Thesis).

ANGELO, M.J. & BISCHOFF, K.B. (1982) A physiologically based pharmacokinetic model for 2,5-hexanedione. In: Proceedings of the 12th Conference on Environmental Toxicology, 1981, Dayton, Ohio, Aerospace Medical Research Laboratory, pp. 250-286 (Paper No. 16) (AFAMRL-TR-81-149).

ANTHONY, D.C., BOEKELHEIDE, K., & GRAHAM, D.G. (1983) The effect of 3,4-dimethyl substitution on the neurotoxicity of 2,5-hexanedione. I. Accelerated clinical neuropathy is accompanied by more proximal axonal swellings. Toxicol. appl. Pharmacol., 71: 362-371.

API (1978) 26 week inhalation toxicity study of n-hexane in the rat, Washington, DC, American Petroleum Institute (API Medical Research Report No. 28-30077).

API (1983a) Six month continuous inhalation exposures of rats to hexane mixtures - phase I, Washington, DC, American Petroleum Institute (API Medical Research Publication No. 30-32858).

API (1983b) Six month continuous inhalation exposures of rats to hexane mixtures - phase II, Washington, DC, American Petroleum Institute (API Medical Research Publication No. 30-32846).

ATKINSON, R., ASCHMANN, S.M., CARTER, W.P.L., WINER, A.M., & PITTS, J.N., Jr (1982) Kinetics of the reactions of OH radicals with n-alkanes at 299 ± 2 K. Int. J. chem. Kinet., 14: 781-788.

BABANOV, G.P. & BABANOV, A.G. (1981) [Permeability of tissues to alkanes and their relationship with molecular weight, parity of carbon atoms and branching of hydrocarbon chains.] Gig. Tr. prof. Zabol., 12: 48-51 (in Russian).

BABANOV, G.P., ABRAMYAN, G.G., ARTEMYEVA, G.N., VERKHOVSKI, L.G., & SHAINA, V.K. (1988) [Elevated temperature effect on animals' sensitivity to n-pentane, n-hexane, n-heptane, n-octane and toluene and their distribution in the tissues.] Gig. Tr. prof. Zabol., 10: 23-25 (in Russian).

BABICH, H., DAVIS, D.L., & ADLER, R. (1982) Updating federal standards for toxicants: n-hexane as the model. Environ. Monit. Assess., 2: 287-299.

BAKER, T.S. & RICKERT, D.E. (1981) Dose-dependent uptake, distribution and elimination of inhaled n-hexane in the Fischer-344 rat. Toxicol. appl. Pharmacol., 61: 414-422.

BAKER, T.S., WHITE, E.L., & RICKERT, D.E. (1980) Differences in the metabolism of n-hexane in Fischer 344 rats and C57B1 mice. Pharmacologist, 22: 279.

BARLOTTA, F., MALFITANO, D., GORGONE, G., & INSERRA, A. (1972) [Electroretinographic study in experimental hexane intoxication.] Boll. Soc. Ital. Biol. Sper., 48: 115-117 (in Italian).

BARNI-COMPARINI, I., LUNGARELLA, G., & FONZI, L. (1982) Responses of lung enzyme activities in rabbits following short-term exposure to n-hexane: correlation between morphological and biochemical changes. Agents Actions, 12: 737-742.

BARTOLUCCI, G.B., MAZZOTTA, M., MANNO, M., & DEROSA, E. (1977) [Industrial exposure to TOCP and n-hexane: behaviour of serum cholinesterase.] Med. Lav., 68: 222-231 (in Italian).

BASTONE, A., FRONTALI, N., MALLOZZI, C., SBRACCIA, M., & SETTIMI, L. (1987) Cholinesterases in blood plasma and tissues of rats treated with n-hexane or with its neurotoxic metabolite 2,4-hexanedione. Arch. Toxicol., 61: 138-144.

BATTISTINI, N., LENZI, G.L., ZANETTE, E., FIESCHI, C., BATTISTA, F., FRANZINELLI, A., & SARTORELLI, E. (1974) [Observations of a group of cases of glue polyneuropathy (Clinical electromyographic and experimental contribution).] Riv. Patol. nerv. ment., 95: 871-885 (in Italian).

BATTISTINI, N., CIONI, R., LENZI, G.L., & ZANETTE, E., (1975) [Study of the H-reflex in glue neuropathy.] Riv. Neurol., 45: 74-79 (in Italian).

BEHNKE, W., HOLLANDER, W., KOCH, W., NOLTING, F., & ZETZSCH, C. (1988) A smog chamber for studies of the photochemical degradation of chemicals in the presence of aerosols. Atmos. Environ., 22: 1113-1120.

BERGER, M.L. & SOZERI, T. (1987) Rapid halogenated hydrocarbon toxicity in isolated hepatocytes is mediated by direct solvent effects. Toxicology, 45: 319-330.

BERNARD, A.M., DE RUSSIS, R., NORMAND, J.-C., & LAUWERYS, R.R. (1989) Evaluation of the subacute nephrotoxicity of cyclohexane and other industrial solvents in the female Sprague-Dawley rat. Toxicol. Lett., 45: 271-280.

BOBRA, A.M., WAN, Y.S., & MACKAY, D. (1983) A predictive correlation for the acute toxicity of hydrocarbons and chlorinated hydrocarbons to the water flea (Daphnia magna). Chemosphere, 12: 1121-1129.

BOCK, F.G. & CHORTYK, O.T. (1970) Tumor promoting activity of aliphatic hydrocarbons. Proc. Am. Assoc. Cancer Res., 11: 9.

BOEKELHEIDE, K. (1987) 2,5-Hexanedione alters microtubule assembly. 1. Testicular atrophy, not nervous system toxicity, correlates with enhanced tubulin polymerization. Toxicol. appl. Pharmacol., 88: 379-382.

BOEKELHEIDE, K. (1988a) Rat testis during 2,5-hexanedione intoxication and recovery. I. Dose response and the reversibility of germ cell loss. Toxicol. appl. Pharmacol., 92: 18-27.

BOEKELHEIDE, K. (1988b) Rat testis during 2,5-hexanedione intoxication and recovery. II. Dynamics of pyrrole reactivity, tubulin content and microtubule assembly. Toxicol. appl. Pharmacol., 92: 28-33.

BOEKELHEIDE, K. & EVELETH, J. (1988) The rate of 2,5-hexanedione intoxication, not total dose, determines the extent of testicular injury and altered micro-tubule assembly in the rat. Toxicol. appl. Pharmacol., 94: 76-83.

BOHLEN, P., SCHLUNEGGER, U.P., & LAUPPI, E. (1973) Uptake and distribution of hexane in rat tissues. Toxicol. appl. Pharmacol., 25: 242-249.

BORGATTI, A.R., TRIGARI, G., VENTRELLA, V., & PAGLIARANI, A. (1981) [Interactions of n-alkanes with respiration and oxidative phosphorylation of rabbit cardiac mitochondria: n-hexane.] Boll. Soc. Ital. Biol. Sper., 56: 1569-1575 (in Italian).

BRAIER, L. (1973) A comparative study of isocyclic hydrocarbons in animals and in man. Haemalogica, 58: 491-500.

BRAVACCIO, F., AMMENDOLA, A., BARRUFFO, L., & CARLOMANGO, S. (1981) H-reflex behaviour in glue (n-hexane) neuropathy. Clin. Toxicol., 18: 1369-1375.

BRINGMANN, G. & KUHN, R. (1982) Results of toxic action of water pollutants on *Daphnia magna* tested by an improved standardized procedure. Z. Wasser Abwasser Forsch., 15: 1-6.

BRUGNONE, F. & PERBELLINI, L. (1980) [Pollution by solvents and workers' positions in shoe and shoe upper factories.] Med. Lav., 71: 343-352 (in Italian).

BRUGNONE, F., PERBELLINI, L., GRIGOLINI, L., & APOSTOLI, P. (1978) Solvent exposure in a shoe upper factory. I. n-Hexane and acetone concen-trations in alveolar and environmental air and in blood. Int. Arch. occup. environ. Health, 42: 51-62.

BRUGNONE, F., PERBELLINI, L., GAFFURI, E., & APOSTOLI, P. (1980) Biomonitoring of industrial solvent exposures in workers' alveolar air. Int. Arch. occup. environ. Health, 47: 245-261.

BRUGNONE, F., PERBELLINI, L., & APOSTOLI, P. (1984) Blood concentration of solvents in industrial exposure. Collect. Méd. lég. Toxicol. méd., 125(Part 1): 165-168.

BUITATTI, E., CECCHINI, S., RONCHI, O., DOLARA, P., & BULGARELLI, G. (1978) Relationship between clinical and electromyographic findings and exposure to solvents, in shoe and leather workers. Br. J. ind. Med., 35: 168-173.

BUS, J.S. & TYL, R.W. (1979) Perinatal toxicity of n-hexane in Fischer 344 rats. Teratology, 19: 22A.

BUS, J.S., WHITE, E.L., TYL, R.W., & BARROW, C.S. (1979) Perinatal toxicity and metabolism of n-hexane in Fischer-344 rats after inhalation exposure during gestation. Toxicol. appl. Pharmacol., 51: 295-302.

BUS, J.S., WHITE, E.L., GILLIES, P.J., & BARROW, C.S. (1981) Tissue distribution of n-hexane, methyl n-butyl ketone and 2,5-hexanedione in rats after single or repeated inhalation exposure to n-hexane. Drug Metab. Dispos., 9: 386-387.

BUS, J.S., DEYO, D., & COX, M. (1982) Dose-dependent disposition of n-hexane in F-344 rats after inhalation exposure. Fundam. appl. Toxicol., 2: 226-229.

CCOHS (1985) n-Hexane, Hamilton, Ontario, Canadian Centre for Occupational Health and Safety (Chemical Hazard Summary No. 11).

CARAPELLA, C. (1977) [Preventive aspects of toxic polyneuropathy in shoe-makers.] Ann. Ist. Super. Sanità, 13: 353-366 (in Italian).

CARLOMAGNO, S., D'ANGELI, A., & MENEGOZZO, M. (1983) [n-Hexane poly-neuropathy in the shoe making and leather industries.] Med. Lav., 74: 111-122 (in Italian).

CAVANAGH, J.B. (1982) The pattern of recovery of axons in the nervous system of rats following 2,5-hexane-diol intoxication. A question of rheology? Neuropathol. appl. Neurobiol., 8: 19-34.

CAVANAGH, J.B. & BENNETTS, R.J. (1981) On the pattern of changes in the nervous system produced by 2,5-hexanediol. A topographical study by light microscopy. Brain, 104: 297-318.

CAVENDER, F.L., CASEY, H.W., SALEM, H., GRAHAM, D.G., SWENBERG, J., & GRALLA, E.J. (1984) A 13-week vapour inhalation study of n-hexane in rats with emphasis on neurotoxic effects. Fundam. appl. Toxicol., 4: 191-201.

CEC (1979) Analysis of organic micropollutants in water, 3rd ed., Luxembourg, Commission of the European Communities, Vol. 1, p. 155 (COST 646 bis).

CHANG, Y.C. (1985) Evoked potential study in n-hexane polyneuropathy. J. Neurol., 22(Suppl.): 200.

CHANG, Y.C. (1987) Neurotoxic effects of n-hexane on the human central nervous system: evoked potential abnormalities in n-hexane polyneuropathy. J. Neurol. Neurosurg. Psychiatry, 50: 269-274.

CHANG, Y.C. & YIP, P.K. (1987) N-hexane-induced electroneurographic changes and early detection of n-hexane intoxication. J. Formosan Med. Assoc., 86: 194-200.

CHAPIN, R.E., NORTON, R.M., POPP, J.A., & BUS, J.S. (1982) The effects of 2,5-hexanedione on reproductive hormones and testicular enzyme activities in the F-344 rat. Toxicol. appl. Pharmacol., 62: 262-272.

CHAPIN, R.E., MORGAN, K.T., & BUS, J.S. (1983) The morphogenesis of testicular degeneration induced in rats by orally administered 2,5-hexanedione. Exp. mol. Pathol., **38**: 149-169.

CHAUPLANNAZ, G., BADY, B., KOPP, N., LEVRAT, R., & TRILLET, M. (1982) Neuropathie périphérique au n-hexane chez une toxicomane. Rev. neurol. (Paris), **138**(3): 249-257.

CHIOU, C.T., KILE, D.E., & MALCOLM, R.L. (1988) Sorption of vapours of some organic liquids on soil humic acid and its relation to partitioning of organic compounds in soil organic matter. Environ. Sci. Technol., **22**: 298-303.

CIANCHETTI, C., ABBRITTI, G. PERTICONI, G., SIRACUSA, A., & CURRADI, F. (1976) Toxic polyneuropathy of shoe industry workers. J. Neurol. Neurosurg. Psychiatry, **39**: 1151-1161.

CIIT (1977) n-Hexane, Research Triangle Park, North Carolina, Chemical Industry Institute of Toxicology (CIIT Current Status Reports, No. 1).

CLAYTON, G.D. & CLAYTON, F.E. (1981) Patty's industrial hygiene and toxicology, New York, Chichester, Brisbane, Toronto, John Wiley and Sons, Vol. 2B.

CFR (1987a) Food additives permitted for direct addition to food for human consumption. Code fed. Regul., 21(Part 172): 172.560, 172.894.

CFR (1987b) Listing of color additives exempt from certification: Subpart B-Drugs. Code fed. Regul., 21(Part 73): 256.

COOPER, R., NEWTON, P., & REED, M. (1985) Neurophysiological signs of brain damage due to glue sniffing. Electroencephalogr. clin. Neurophysiol., **60**: 23-26.

COURI, D. & MILKS, M. (1982) Toxicity and metabolism of the neurotoxic hexacarbons n-hexane, 2-hexanone and 2,5-hexanedione. Annu. Rev. Pharmacol. Toxicol., **22**: 145-166.

COURI, D., ABDEL-RAHMAN, M.S., & HETLAND, L.B. (1978) Biotransformation of n-hexane and methyl n-butyl ketone in guinea pigs and mice. Am. Ind. Hyg. Assoc. J., **39**: 295-300.

CREPET, M., GAFFURI, E., & PICOTTI, G. (1968) [Triarylphosphate disease in the shoe industry.] Minerva med., **59**(78): 4073-4075 (in Italian).

DAHL, A.R., DAMON, E.G., MAUDERLY, J.L., ROTHENBERG, S.J., SEILER, F.A., & MCCLELLAN, R.O. (1988) Uptake of 19 hydrocarbon vapors inhaled by F344 rats. Fundam. appl. Toxicol., **10**: 262-269.

DALE, G.H. & DREHMAN, L.E. (1985) Hexane. In: Kirk-Othmer encyclopedia of chemical technology, 3rd ed., New York, Chichester, Brisbane, Toronto, John Wiley and Sons, pp 926-930.

DECAPRIO, A.P. (1987) n-Hexane neurotoxicity: A mechanism involving pyrrole adduct formation in axonal cytoskeletal protein. Neurotoxicology, **8**: 199-210.

DECAPRIO, A.P. & O'NEILL, E.A. (1985) Alterations in rat axonal cytoskeletal proteins induced by *in vitro* and *in vivo* 2,5-hexanedione exposure. Toxicol. appl. Pharmacol., **78**: 235-247.

DECAPRIO, A.P., OLAJOS, E.J., & WEBER, P. (1982) Covalent binding of a neurotoxic n-hexane metabolite: conversion of primary amines to substituted pyrrole adducts by 2,5-hexanedione. Toxicol. appl. Pharmacol., **65**: 440-450.

DECAPRIO, A.P., BRIGSS, R.G., JACKOWSKI, S.J., & KIM, J.C.S. (1988) Comparative neurotoxicity and pyrrole-forming potential of 2,5-hexanedione and perdenterio-2.5-hexanedione in the rat. Toxicol. appl. Pharmacol., **92**: 75-85.

DE GROOT, D.M.G. & KEPNER, L.A. (1984) The effects of long term discontinuous exposure to low levels of n-hexane on rats, Zeist, The Netherlands, Medical Biological Laboratory, TNO (Conducted on behalf of Shell Internationale Petroleum Maatschappij BV).

DEICHMANN, W.B. & LE BLANC, T.J. (1943) Determination of the approximate lethal dose with about six animals. J. ind. Hyg. Toxicol., **25**: 415-417.

DELBRÜCK, W.R. & KLUGE, A. (1982) [The effects of n-hexane in man and animals], Hamburg, German Society for Petroleum Sciences and Coal Chemistry (Research Report No. 174-2) (in German).

DEMARTINO, C., MALORNI, W., AMANTINI, M.C., SCORZA BARCELLONA, P., & FRONTALI, N. (1987) Effects of respiratory treatment with n-hexane on rat testis morphology. I. A light microscope study. Exp. mol. Pathol., **46**: 199-216.

DE ROSA, E., BARTOLUCCI, G.B., PERBELLINI, L., BRUGNONE, F., & RAUSA, G. (1988) Environmental and biological monitoring of exposure to toluene, styrene and n-hexane. Appl. ind. Hyg., **3**: 332-337.

DFG (Deutsche Forschungsgemeinschaft) (1988) Maximum concentrations at the workplace and biological tolerance values for working materials: Report No. XXIV of the Commission for the Investigation of Health Hazards of Chemical Compounds in the Work Area, Weinheim, Verlag Chemie, p. 84.

DI-BOSCO, M. & FONZI, S. (1974) [So-called glue or shoe makers' polyneuropathy.] Riv. Infort. Mal. prof., **61**(Part 1): 165-192 (in Italian).

DISCALZI, G.L., PERRELLI, G., & PAVAN, I. (1988) [Solvent exposure risk among homeworkers.] Med. Lav., **79**: 234-236 (in Italian).

DIVINCENZO, G.D., KAPLAN, C.J., & DEDINAS, J. (1976) Characterization of the metabolites of methyl n-butyl ketone, methyl isobutyl ketone and methyl ethyl ketone in guinea pig serum and their clearance. Toxicol. appl. Pharmacol., **36**: 511-522.

DIVINCENZO, G.D., HAMILTON, M.L., KAPLAN, C.J., & DEDINAS, J. (1977) Metabolic fate and disposition of ^{14}C-labelled methyl n-butyl ketone in the rat. Toxicol. appl. Pharmacol., **41**: 547-560.

DIVINCENZO, G.D., HAMILTON, M.L., KAPLAN, C.J., KRASAVAGE, W.J., & O'DONOGHUE, J.L. (1978) Studies on the respiratory uptake and excretion and the skin absorption of methyl n-butyl ketone in humans and dogs. Toxicol. appl. Pharmacol., 44: 593-604.

DIVINCENZO, G.D., KRASAVAGE, W.J., & O'DONOGHUE, J.L. (1980) Role of metabolism in hexacarbon neuropathy. In: Witschi, H., ed. The scientific basis of toxicity assessment, Amsterdam, Oxford, New York, Elsevier Science Publishers, pp. 183-200.

DOLARA, P., FRANCONI, F., & BASOSI, D. (1978) Urinary excretion of some n-hexane metabolites. Pharmacol. Res. Commun., 10(6): 503-510.

DUNNICK, J.K. (1989) Toxicity studies of n-hexane in B6C3F, mice (inhalation studies), Washington, DC, US Department of Health and Human Services, National Toxicology Program (Report No. NTPTS 1).

DUNNICK, J.K., GRAHAM, D.G., YANG, R.S.H., HABER, S.B., & BROWN, H.R. (1989) Thirteen-week toxicity study of n-hexane in B6C3F, mice after inhalation exposure. Toxicology, 57: 163-172.

DURHAM, H.D., PENA, S.D.J., & CARPENTER, S. (1983) The neurotoxins 2,5-hexanedione and acrylamide promote aggregation in intermediate filaments in cultured fibroblasts. Muscle Nerve, 6: 631-637.

DURHAM, H.D., PENA, S.D.J., & ECOBICHON, D.J. (1988) Hexahydrocarbon effects on intermediate filament organization in human fibroblasts. Muscle Nerve, 11: 160-165.

EBEN, A., FLUCKE, W., MINAIL, F., THYSSEN, J., & KIMMERLE, G. (1979) Toxicological and metabolic studies of methyl n-butyl ketone, 2,5-hexanedione and 2,5-hexanediol in male rats. Ecotoxicol. environ. Saf., 3: 204-217.

EDELFORS, S. & RAVN-JONSEN, A. (1985) Calcium uptake in rat brain synaptomsomes after short-term exposure to organic solvents: a pilot study. Acta pharmacol. toxicol., 56: 431-434.

ELKINS, H.B. (1959) The chemistry of industrial toxicology, 2nd ed., New York, Chichester, Brisbane, Toronto, John Wiley and Sons.

FAWCETT, P.R.W. & BARWICK, D.D. (1981) Studies in nerve conduction. In: Walton, J.A., ed. Disorders of voluntary muscle, 4th ed., New York, Churchill Livingstone, pp. 928-951.

FEDTKE, N. & BOLT, H.M. (1986a) Detection of 2,5-hexanedione in the urine of persons not exposed to n-hexane. Int. Arch. occup. environ. Health, 57: 143-148.

FEDTKE, N. & BOLT, H.M. (1986b) Methodological investigations on the determination of n-hexane metabolites in urine. Int. Arch. occup. environ. Health, 57: 149-158.

FEDTKE, N. & BOLT, H.M. (1987a) 4,5-dihydroxy-2-hexanone: a new metabolite of n-hexane and of 2,5-hexanedione in rat urine. Biochem. environ. mass Spectrom., 14: 563-572.

FEDTKE, N. & BOLT, H.M. (1987b) The relevance of 4,5-dihydroxy-2-hexanone in the excretion kinetics of n-hexane metabolites in rat and man. Arch. Toxicol., 61: 131-137

FICHERA, G., SPAGNA, C., & TIMPANARO, V. (1968) [Hydrocarbon intoxication. Note II. Anatomo-pathological findings in experimental hexane intoxication.] Folia med. (Napoli), 51: 633-640 (in Italian).

FILSER, J.G., PETER, H., BOLT, H.M., & FEDTKE, N. (1987) Pharmacokinetics of the neurotoxin n-hexane in rat and man. Arch. Toxicol., 60: 77-80.

FISEROVA-BERGEROVA, V. & PIERCE, J.T. (1989) Biological monitoring V: Dermal absorption. Appl. ind. Hyg., 8(4): F14-F21.

FRANCHINI, I., CAVATORTA, A., FALZOI, M., LUCERTINI, S., & MUTTI, A. (1983) Early indicators of renal damage in workers exposed to organic solvents. Int. Arch. occup. environ. Health, 52: 1-9.

FRANKE, J.P., WIJSBEEK, J., DE ZEEUZ, R.A., MOLLER, M.R., & NIERMEYER, H. (1988) Systematic analysis of solvents and other volatile substances by gas chromatography. J. anal. Toxicol., 12: 20-24.

FROMMER, U., ULLRICH, V., & ORRENIUS, S. (1974) Influence of inducers and inhibitors on the hydroxylation pattern of n-hexane in rat liver microsomes. FEBS Lett., 41(1): 14-16.

FRONTALI, N., AMANTINI, M.C., SPAGNOLO, A., GUARCINI, A.M., & SALTARI, M.C. (1981) Experimental neurotoxicity and urinary metabolites of the C5-C7 alphatic hydrocarbons used as glue solvents in shoe manufacture. Clin. Toxicol., 18(12): 1357-1367.

FUHNER, H. (1921) [The narcotic effects of gasoline and its components (pentane, hexane, heptane, octane).] Biochem. Z., 115: 235-261 (in German).

GENTER, M.B., SZAKAL-QUIN, G., ANDERSON, C.W., ANTHONY, D.C., & GRAHAM, D.G. (1987) Evidence that pyrrole formation is a pathogenetic step in γ-diketone neuropathy. Toxicol. appl. Pharmacol., 87: 351-361.

GENTER ST. CLAIR, M.B., AMARNATH, V., MOODY, A., ANTHONY, D.C., ANDERSON, C.W., & GRAHAM, D.G. (1988) Pyrrole oxidation and protein cross-linking as necessary steps in the development of γ-diketone neuropathy. Chem. Res. Toxicol., 1: 179-185.

GENTRY, S.J. & WALSH, P.T. (1987) Eight-hour TWA personal monitoring using a diffusive sampler and short-term stain tube. Am. Ind. Hyg. Assoc. J., 48: 287-292.

GERARDE, H.W. & LINDEN, N.J. (1963) Toxicological studies on hydrocarbons. IX. The aspiration hazard and toxicity of hydrocarbons and hydrocarbon mixtures. Arch. environ. Health, 6: 329-341.

GHITTORI, S., IMBRIANI, M., PEZZAGNO, G., & CAPODAGLIO, E. (1987) The urinary concentration of solvents as a biological indicator of exposure: proposal for the biological equivalent exposure limit for nine solvents. Am. Ind. Hyg. Assoc. J., **48**: 786-790.

GILLIES, P.J., NORTON, R.M., WHITE, E.L., & BUS, J.S. (1980) Inhibition of sciatic nerve sterologenesis in hexacarbon-induced distal axonopathy in the rat. Toxicol. appl. Pharmacol., **54**: 217-222.

GIULIANO, G., IANNACCONE, A., & ZAPPOLI, R. (1974) [Electroencephalographic research in shoe industry workers exposed to the risk of poisoning from adhesive solvents.] Lav. Um., 26(2): 33-42 (in Italian).

GOEL, S.K., RAO, G.S., & PANDYA, K.P. (1982) Toxicity of n-hexane and n-heptane: some biochemical changes in liver and serum. Toxicol. Lett., **14**: 169-174.

GOEL, S.K., RAO, G.S., & KRISHNAMURTI, C.R. (1987) Toxicity of n-hexane and 2,5-hexanediol to the haemopoietic system: a preliminary report. Xenobiotica, **17**: 217-222.

GOEL, S.K., RAO, G.S., & PANDYA, K.P. (1988) Hepatotoxic effects elicited by n-hexane or n-heptane. J. appl. Toxicol., **8**: 81-84.

GOMEZ-ARROYO, S., CASTILLO-RUIZ, P., & VILLALOBOS-PIETRINI, R. (1986) Chromosomal alterations induced in *Vicia faba* by different industrial solvents: thinner, toluene, benyene, n-hexane, n-heptane and ethyl acetate. Cytologia, **51**: 133-142.

GONZALEZ, E.G. & DOWNEY, J.A. (1972) Polyneuropathy in a glue sniffer. Arch. phys. Med. Rehabil., **53**: 333-337.

GOTO, I., MATSUMURA, M., INOUE, N., MURAI, Y., SHIDA, K., SANTA, T., & KUROIWA, Y. (1974) Toxic polyneuropathy due to glue sniffing. J. Neurol. Neurosurg. Psychiatry, **37**: 848-853.

GRAHAM, D.G. & GOTTFREID, M.R. (1984) Cross species extrapolation in hydrocarbon neuropathy. Neurobehav. Toxicol. Teratol., **6**: 433-435.

GRAHAM, D.G., ANTHONY, D.C., & BOEKELHEIDE, K. (1982a) *In vitro* and *in vivo* studies of the molecular pathogenesis of n-hexane neuropathy. Neurobehav. Toxicol. Teratol., **4**: 629-634.

GRAHAM, D.G., ANTHONY, D.C., BOEKELHEIDE, K., MASCHMANN, N.A., RICHARDS, R.G., WOLFRAM, J.W., & SHAW, B.R. (1982b) Studies of the molecular pathogenesis of hexane neuropathy. II. Evidence that pyrrole derivatization of lysyl residues leads to protein crosslinking. Toxicol. appl. Pharmacol., **64**: 415-422.

GRAHAM, D.G., ANTHONY, D.C., SZAKAL-QUIN, G., GOTTFREID, M.R., & BOEKELHEIDE, K. (1985) Covalent crosslinking of neurofilaments in the pathogenesis of n-hexane neuropathy. Neurotoxicology, **6**: 55-64.

GRIFFITHS, I.R., KELLY, P.A.T., CARMICHAEL, S., MCCULLOCH, M., & WATERSON, M. (1981) The relationship of glucose utilization and morphological change in the visual system in hexacarbon neuropathy. Brain Res., 222: 447-451.

GRIFFITH, J.F., NIXON, G.A., BRUCE, R.D., REER, P.J., & BANNAN, E.A. (1980) Dose-response studies with chemical irritants in the albino rabbit eye as a basis for selecting optimum testing conditions for predicting hazard to the human eye. Toxicol. appl. Pharmacol., 55: 501-513.

GOVERNA, M., CALISTI, R., COPPA, G., TAGLIAVENTO, G., COLOMBI, A., & TRONI, W. (1987) Urinary excretion of 2,5-hexanedione and peripheral polyneuropathies in workers exposed to hexane. J. Toxicol. environ. Health, 20: 219-228.

GROVES, F.R. (1988) Effect of cosolvents on the solubility of hydrocarbons in water. Environ. Sci. Technol., 22: 282-286.

GUTHRIE, V.B. (1960) Petroleum products handbook, New York, McGraw-Hill.

HADJIIVANOVA, N.B., SALOVSKI, P.Z., GROSEVA, M.M., CHARAKCHIEVA, S.B., & NECHEV, Ch.K. (1987) Early effects of n-hexane and irradiation on the lung surfactant system. Acta physiol. pharmacol. Bulg., 13: 25-29.

HAZELTON LABORATORIES (1981) In vivo and in vitro mutagenicity studies n-hexane (hexane UV), Vienna, Virginia, Hazelton Laboratories (Project No. 596-114 and 596-115) (Prepared for the American Petroleum Institute).

HENDERSON, V.E. & SMITH, A.H.R. (1936) Propylene impurities. Hexenes and hexanes. J. Pharmacol. exp. Ther., 58: 319-327.

HERSKOWITZ, A., ISHII, N., & SCHAUMBERG, H. (1971) n-Hexane neuropathy. A syndrome occurring as a result of industrial exposure. New Engl. J. Med., 285(2): 82-85.

HEWITT, W.R., MIYAJIMA, H., COTE, M., & PLAA, G.L. (1980) Acute alteration of chloroform induced hepato- and nephrotoxicity by n-hexane, methyl n-butyl ketone and 2,5-hexanedione. Toxicol. appl. Pharmacol., 53: 230-248.

HINE, C.H. & ZUIDEMA, H.H. (1970) The toxicological properties of hydrocarbon solvents. Ind. Med., 39(5): 39-44.

HODGSON, A.T., GIRMAN, J.R., & BINENBOYM, J. (1986) A multisorbent sampler for volatile organic compounds in indoor air. In: Proceedings of the 79th Annual Meeting, Minneapolis, 22-27 June, 1986, Minneapolis, Minnesota, Air Pollution Control Association, pp. 1-15 (Report No. 86-37-1).

HOLMBERG, B. & LUNDBERG, P. (1989) Assessment and management of occupational risks in the Nordic (Scandinavian) countries. Am. J. ind. Med., 15: 615-626.

HONMA, T. (1983) Changes in acetylcholine metabolism in rat brain after a short-term exposure to toluene and n-hexane. Toxicol. Lett., 16: 17-22.

HONMA, T., MIYAGAWA, M., SATO, M., & HASEGAWA, H. (1982) Increase in glutamine content of rat midbrain induced by short-term exposure to toluene and hexane. Ind. Health, 20: 109-115.

HOUK, V.S., SCHALKOWSKY, S., & CLAXTON, L.D. (1989) Development and validation of the spiral Salmonella assay: an automated approach to bacterial mutagenicity testing. Mutat. Res., 223: 49-64.

HOWD, R.A., BINGHAM, L.R., STEEGER, T.M., REBERT, C.S., & PRYOR, G.T. (1982) Relation between schedules of exposure to hexane and plasma levels of 2,5-hexanedione. Neurobehav. Toxicol. Teratol., 4: 87-91.

HOWD, R.A., REBERT, C.S., DICKINSON, J., & PRYOR, G. (1983) A comparison of the rates of development of functional hexane neuropathy in weanling and young adult rats. Neurobehav. Toxicol. Teratol., 5: 63-68.

HOWELL, W.E. (1979) A neurobehavioural evaluation of the pre-natal toxicity of n-hexane in rats, Cincinnati, Ohio, University of Ohio, 78 pp (Ph.D Thesis) (Dissertation Abstracts Int B. No. 1610B).

HOWELL, W.E. & COOPER, G.P. (1981) Neurophysiological evaluation of prenatal n-hexane toxicity. Toxicologist, 1: 152 (Abstact 552).

HUANG, C.-C. & CHU, N.-S. (1989) Evoked potentials in chronic n-hexane intoxication. Clin. Electroencephalogr., 20: 162-168.

HUSMAN, K. & KARLI, P. (1980) Clinical neurological findings among car painters exposed to a mixture of organic solvents. Scand. J. Work Environ. Health, 6: 33-39.

ICHIHARA, K., KUSONOSE, E., & KUSUNOSE, M. (1969) Microsomal hydroxylation of decane. Biochem. Biophys. Acta, 176: 713-719.

IIDA, M. (1982) Neurophysiological studies of n-hexane polyneuropathy in the sandal factory. Electroencephalogr. clin. Neurophysiol., 36(Suppl.): 671-681.

IIDA, M. & YAMAMOTO, H. (1973) [Prognosis of n-hexane polyneuropathy. Follow-up studies of mass outbreak in District F in Mie Prefecture.] Igaku Ayumi, 84(4): 199-201 (in Japanese).

IIDA, M., YAMAMURA, Y., & SOBUE, I. (1969) Electromyographical findings and conduction velocity in n-hexane polyneuropathy. Electromyography, 9: 247-261.

IKEDA, M. & KASAHARA, M. (1986) n-Hexane and benzene contents in gasolene for industrial purpose. Ind. Health, 24: 63-66.

IKEDA, M., KOIZUMI, A., KASAHARA, M., & FUJITA, H. (1986) Combined effects of n-hexane and toluene on norepinephrine and dopamine levels in rat brain tissues after long-term exposures. Bull. environ. Contam. Toxicol., 36: 510-517.

IMBRIANI, M., GHITTORI, S., BORLINI, F., PEZZAGNO, G., & CAPODAGLIO, E. (1984a) [n-Hexane and toluene in the urine of occupationally exposed subjects.] Boll. Soc. Ital. Biol. Sper., 60: 1919-1925 (in Italian).

IMBRIANI, M., GHITTORI, S., PEZZAGNO, G., & CAPODAGLIO, E. (1984b) n-Hexane urine elimination and weighted exposure concentration. Int. Arch. occup. environ. Health, 55: 33-41.

INOUE, T., TAKEUCHI, Y., TAKEUCHI, S., YAMADA, S., SUZUKI, H., MATSUSHITA, T., MIYAGAKI, M., MAEDA, K., & MATSUMOTO, T. (1970) [Industrial health survey of high incidence of n-hexane intoxication among vinyl sandal manufacturers.] Ind. Health, 12(3): 73-84 (in Japanese).

INOUE, T., YAMADA, S., MIYAGAKI, H., & TAKEUCHI, Y. (1971) Polyneuritis caused by n-hexane and the maximum allowable concentration. In: Proceedings of the XVI International Congress on Occupational Health, 22-27 September 1969, Tokyo, Industrial Safety Association, pp. 522-524.

IRPTC (1990) IRPTC Legal file, Geneva, International Register of Potentially Toxic Chemicals, United Nations Environment Programme.

ISHIDATE, M. & SOFUNI, T. (1984) Primary mutagenicity screening of food additives currently used in Japan. Food chem. Toxicol., 22(8): 623-636.

IWASAKI, K. & TSURUTA, H. (1984) Molecular mechanisms of hexane neuropathy. Significant differences in pharmacokinetics between 2,3- 2,4-, and 2,5-hexanedione. Ind. Health, 22: 177-187.

IWATA, M., TAKEUCHI, Y., HISANAGA, N., & ONO, Y. (1983a) Changes of n-hexane metabolites in urine of rats exposed to various concentrations of n-hexane and to its mixture with toluene or MEK. Int. Arch. occup. environ. Health, 53: 1-8.

IWATA, M., TAKEUCHI, Y., HISANAGA, N., & ONO, Y. (1983b) A study on biological monitoring of n-hexane exposure. Int. Arch. occup. environ. Health, 51: 253-260.

IWATA, M., TAKEUCHI, Y., HISANAGA, N., & ONO, Y. (1984) Changes of n-hexane neurotoxicity and its urinary metabolites by long-term co-exposure with MEK or toluene. Int. Arch. occup. environ. Health, 54: 273-281.

JAKOBSON, I., WAHLBERG, J.E., HOLMBERG, B., & JOHANSSON, G. (1982) Uptake via the blood and elimination of 10 organic solvents following epicutaneous exposure of anaesthetized guinea pigs. Toxicol. appl. Pharmacol., 63: 181-187.

JEPPSSON, R. (1975) Parabolic relationship between lipophilicity and biological activity of aliphatic hydrocarbons, ethers and ketones after intravenous injection of emulsion formulations into mice. Acta pharmacol. toxicol., 37: 56-64.

JONES, H.G. & CAVANAGH, J.B. (1982) Recovery from 2,5-hexanediol intoxication of the retinotectal tract of the rat. An ultrastructural study. Acta neuropathol. (Berlin), 58: 286-290.

JUHNKE, I. & LUDEMANN, D. (1978) [Results of trials of 200 chemical compounds for acute toxicity for fish with the golden orfe test.] Z. Wasser Abwasser Forsch., 11: 161-164 (in German).

KANNAN, K., SINGH, K.P., GOEL, S., & SHANKER, R. (1985) Effects of 2,5-hexanedione on immunocompetence of mice. Environ. Res., **36**: 14-25.

KASAHARA, M. & IKEDA, M. (1987) Spontaneous desorption of organic solvents from carbon cloth. Ind. Health, **25**: 73-81

KASAHARA, M., SUZUKI, H., TAKEUCHI, Y., HARA, I., & IKEDA, M. (1987) n-Hexane, benzene and other aromatic components in petroleum distillate solvents in Japan. Ind. Health, **25**: 205-214.

KATAGIRI, Y. & OHASHI, T. (1975) Photochemical reactions of hydrocarbons in smog chamber. Annu. Rep. Kanagawa Prefect. Environ. Cent., **6**: 47.

KATZ, G.V., O'DONOGHUE, J.L., DIVINCENZO, G.D., & TERHAAR, C.J. (1980) Comparative neurotoxicity and metabolism of ethyl n-butyl ketone and methyl n-butyl ketone in rats. Toxicol. appl. Pharmacol., **52**: 153-158.

KAWACHI, T., YAHAGI, T., KADA, T., TAZIMA, Y., ISHIDATE, M., SASAKI, M., & SUGIYAMA, T. (1982) Co-operative programme on short-term assays for carcinogenicity in Japan. In: Molecular and cellular aspects of carcinogen screening tests, Lyon, International Agency for Research on Cancer, pp. 323-330 (IARC Scientific Publications No. 27).

KEPLINGER, M.L., LANIER, G.E., & DEICHMANN, W.B. (1959) Effects of environmental temperature on the acute toxicity of a number of compounds in rats. Toxicol. appl. Pharmacol., **1**: 156-161.

KIMURA, E.T., EBERT, D.M., & DODGE, P.W. (1971) Acute toxicity and limits of solvent residue for sixteen organic solvents. Toxicol. appl. Pharmacol., **19**: 699-704.

KLIGMAN, A.M. (1966) The identification of contact allergens by human assay. III. The maximization test: a procedure for screening and rating contact sensitisers. J. invest. Dermatol., **47**: 393-409.

KLIMES, I., VISKUPIC, E., ZORAD, S., SVABOVA, E., KISS, A., & MACHO, L. (1987) Effect of prolonged n-hexane administration on *in vitro* insulin degradation in rat liver and blood. Med. Sci. Res., **15**: 1427-1429.

KLOPFFER, W., HAAG, F., KOHL, E.-G., & FRANK, R. (1988) Testing of the abiotic degradation of chemicals in the atmosphere: The smog chamber approach. Ecotoxicol. environ. Saf., **15**: 298-319.

KOROBKIN, R., ASBURY, A.K., SUMNER, A.J., & NIELSEN, S.L., (1975) Glue sniffing neuropathy. Arch. Neurol., **32**: 158-162.

KRÄMER, A., STAUDINGER, H., & ULLRICH, V. (1974) Effect of n-hexane inhalation on the monooxygenase system in mice liver microsomes. Chem.-biol. Interact., **8**: 11-18.

KRASAVAGE, W.J., O'DONOGHUE, J.L., & TERHAAR, C.J. (1979) Oral chronic toxicity of methyl n-propyl ketone, methyl n-butyl ketone and hexane in rats. Toxicol. appl. Pharmacol., **48**(Part 2): A205.

KRASAVAGE, W.J., O'DONOGHUE, J.L., DIVINCENZO, G.D., & TERHAAR, C.J. (1980) The relative neurotoxicity of methyl n-butyl ketone, n-hexane and their metabolites. Toxicol. appl. Pharmacol., 52: 433-441.

KRONEVI, T., WAHLBERG, J., & HOLMBERG., B. (1979) Histopathology of skin, liver and kidney after epicutaneous administration of five industrial solvents to guinea-pigs. Environ. Res., 19: 56-69.

KULIG, B.M. (1983) Chronic behavioural toxicology of hexane and CS2: Progress report, Zeist, The Netherlands, Medical Biological Laboratory, TNO (Conducted on behalf of Shell Internationale Petroleum Maatschappij BV).

KULIG, B.M. & WOLTHIUS, O.L. (1984) The development of neurological and behavioural impairments in rats exposed subchronically to n-hexane. In: Abstracts of the International Conference on Organic Solvent Toxicity, Stockholm, October 1984.

KULIG, B.M., DEMIK, G., & WOLTHIUS, O.L. (1984) 2,5-Hexanedione concentrations and hexane-induced neuropathy in Wistar rats. Abstracts of the Second International Conference on Neurotoxicology of Selected Chemicals, Chicago, 1983. Neurotoxicology, 5(2): 307.

KULIG, B.M., VANWERSCH, R.A.P., & WOLTHUIS, O.L. (1985) The automated analysis of coordinated hindlimb movement in rats during acute and prolonged exposure to toxic agents. Toxicol. appl. Pharmacol., 80: 1-10.

KURITA, H. (1974) [Experimental studies on the effects of n-hexane on albino rats.] Ind. Health, 9(8): 24-29 (in Japanese).

LADEFOGED, O. & PERBELLINI, L. (1986) Acetone-induced changes in the toxicokinetics of 2,5-hexanedione in rabbits. Scand. J. Work. Environ. Health, 12: 627-629.

LADEFOGED, O., HASS, U., & SIMONSEN, L. (1989) Neurophysiological and bahavioural effects of combined exposure to 2,5-hexanedione and acetone or ethanol in rats. Pharmacol. Toxicol., 65: 372-375.

LAFFORT, P. & DRAVNIEKS, A. (1973) An approach to a physico-chemical model of olfactory stimulation in vertebrates by single compounds. J. theor. Biol., 38: 335-345.

LAGUENY, A., JULIEN, J., VALLAT, J.M., FERRER, X., DELIAC, P., & DELIAC, M. (1982) Etude électrophysiologique de deux cas de polynévrite provoquée par une association n-hexane-méthyléthyl-cétone. Rev. EEG Neurophysiol., 12: 158-166.

LANKAS, G.R., BAXTER, C.S., & CHRISTIAN, R.T. (1978) Effect of alkane tumour-promoting agents on chemically induced mutagenesis in cultured V79 Chinese hamster cells. J. Toxicol. environ. Health, 4: 37-41.

LAPADULA, D.M., IRWIN, R., SUWITA, E., & ABOU-DONIA, M.B. (1986) Cross-linking of neurofilament proteins of rat spinal cord *in vivo* after administration of 2,5-hexanedione. J. Neurochem., 46: 1843-1850.

LAZAREV, N.W. (1929) [The toxicity of various hydrocarbon vapours.] Arch. exp. Pathol. Pharmakol., **143**: 223-233 (in German).

LIJINSKY, W. & RAHA, C.R. (1961) Polycyclic aromatic hydrocarbons in commercial solvents. Toxicol. appl. Pharmacol., **3**: 469-473.

LITTON BIONETICS (1979) Teratology study in rats: n-hexane, Litton Bionetics (LBI Project No. 20698-9) (Final Report submitted to the American Petroleum Institute).

LITTON BIONETICS (1980) Mutagenicity evaluation of n-hexane in the mouse dominant lethal assay, Litton Bionetics (LBI Project No. 21141-01) (Final Report submitted to the American Petroleum Institute).

LODEN, M. (1986) The *in vitro* permeability of human skin to benzene, ethylene glycol, formaldehyde and n-hexane. Acta pharmacol. toxicol., **58**: 382-389.

LONNEMAN, W.A., KOPCZYNSKI, S.L., DARLEY, P.E., & SUTTERFIELD, F.D. (1974) Hydrocarbon composition of urban air pollution. Environ. Sci. Technol., **8**: 229-236.

LUNGARELLA, G., FONZI, L., & CENTINI, F. (1980) Respiratory tract lesions induced in rabbits by short-term exposure to n-hexane. Res. Commun. chem. Pathol. Pharmacol., **29**(1): 129-139.

LUNGARELLA, G., BARNI-COMPARINI, I., & FONZI, L. (1984) Pulmonary changes induced in rabbits by long-term exposure to n-hexane. Arch. Toxicol., **55**: 224-228.

MCAULIFFE, C. (1963) Solubility in water of C1-C9 hydrocarbons. Nature (Lond.), **200**: 1092-1093.

MCCARROLL, N.E., PIPER, C.E., & KEECH, B.H., (1980) Bacterial microsuspension assays with benzene and other organic solvents. Environ. Mutagen., **2**(2): 281-281.

MCCARROLL, N.E., PIPER, C.E., & KEECH, B.H. (1981a) An E. coli microsuspension assay for the detection of DNA damage induced by direct-acting agents and promutagens. Environ. Mutagen., **3**: 429-444.

MCCARROLL, N.E., KEECH, B.H., & PIPER, C.E. (1981b) A microsuspension adaptation of the *Bacillus subtilis* "rec" assay. Environ. Mutagen., **3**: 607-616.

MCNAMARA, B.C. & JEFCOATE, C.R. (1988) Synergistic stimulation of pregnenolone synthesis in rat adrenal mitochondria by n-hexane and cardiolipin. Arch. Biochem. Biophys., **260**: 780-788.

MAHMOUD, G. & LACHAPELLE, J.M. (1984) Etude de l'efficacité d'un gel de protection anti-solvants, vis-à-vis de l'irritation cutanée provoquée par le n-hexane. Arch. Mal. prof. Méd. Trav. Séc. soc., **45**(4): 223-237.

MAHMOUD, G. & LACHAPELLE, J.M. (1985) Evaluation expérimentale de l'efficacité de crèmes-barrière et de gels antisolvants dans la prévention de l'irritation cutanée provoquée par des solvants organiques. Cah. Méd. Trav., 22(2/3): 163-168.

MAIZLISH, N.A., LANGOLF, G.D., WHITEHEAD, L.W., FINE, L.J., ALBERS, J.W., GOLDBERG, J., & SMITH, P. (1985) Behavioural evaluation of workers exposed to mixtures of organic solvents. Br. J. ind. Med., 42: 579-590.

MAIZLISH, N.A., FINE, L.J., ALBERS, J.W., WHITEHEAD, L., & LANGOLF, G.D. (1987) A neurological evaluation of workers exposed to mixtures of organic solvents. Br. J. ind. Med., 44: 14-25.

MALORNI, W., DEMARTINO, C., AMANTINI, M., & FRONTALI, N. (1984) Effects of subchronic treatment with n-hexane on rat testis. A morphological study. Ultramicroscopy, 12: 148.

MALORNI, W., FORMISANO, G., & DONELLI, G. (1989) Morphologic changes induced *in vitro* by 2,5-hexanedione. In vitro cell. dev. Biol., 25: 82-90.

MARCHISEPPE, I., VALENTINO, M., GOVERNA, M., & STOCCHI, V. (1989) Determination of total 2,5-hexanedione by reversed-phase high-performance liquid chromatography. J. Chromatology, 495: 288-294.

MARKS, T.A., FISHER, P.W., & STAPLES, R.E. (1980) Influence of n-hexane on embryo and fetal development in mice. Drug chem. Toxicol., 3(4): 393-406.

MELLAN, I., ed. (1977) Industrial solvents handbook, 2nd ed., Park Ridge, New Jersey, Noyes Data Corporation, p. 14.

MEDINILLA, J., DE & ESPIGARES, M. (1989) [Hexane levels in olive dreg extraction plants in Granada, Spain.] Ig. mod., 91: 353-361 (in Spanish).

MISUMI, J. & NAGANO, M. (1984) Neurophysiological studies on the relation between the structural properties and neurotoxicity of aliphatic hydrocarbon compounds in rats. Br. J. ind. Med., 41: 526-532.

MISUMI, J. & NAGANO, M. (1985) Experimental study on the enhancement of the neurotoxicity of methyl butyl ketone by non-neurotoxic aliphatic monoketones. Br. J. ind. Med., 42: 155-161.

MIYAGAKI, H. (1967) [Electrophysiological studies of the peripheral neurotoxicity of n-hexane.] Ind. Health, 9: 660-671 (in Japanese).

MORTELMANS, K., HAWORTH, S., LAWLOR, T., SPECK, W., TAINER, B., & ZEIGER, E. (1986) Salmonella mutagenicity tests. II. Results from the testing of 270 chemicals. Environ. Mutagen., 8(Suppl. 7): 1-119.

MUTTI, A., LUCERTINI, S., VENTURI, G., CAVATORTA, A., & FRANCHINI, I. (1980) Organic solvents and glomerulonephritis. Negative epidemiological findings for hydrocarbons. Abstracts of the 2nd International Congress on Toxicology, Brussels. Toxicol. Lett., Spec. Issue 1: 220.

MUTTI, A., LUCERTINI, S., FALZOI, M., CAVATORTA, A., & FRANCHINI, I. (1981) Organic solvents and chronic glomerulonephritis. A cross-sectional study with negative findings for aliphatic and alicyclic C5-C7 hydrocarbons. J. appl. Toxicol., 1(4): 224-226.

MUTTI, A., CAVATORTA, A., LUCERTINI, S., ARFINI, G., FALZOI, M., & FRANCHINI, I. (1982a) Neurophysiological changes in workers exposed to organic solvents in a shoe factory. Scand. J. Work Environ. Health, 8(Suppl. 1): 136-141.

MUTTI, A., CAVATORTA, A., LOMMI, G., LOTTA, S., & FRANCHINI, I. (1982b) Neurophysiological effect of long term exposure to hydrocarbon mixtures. Arch. Toxicol., Suppl. 5: 120-124.

MUTTI, A., FERRI, F., LOMMI, G., LOTTA, S., LUCERTINI, S., & FRANCHINI, I. (1982c) n-Hexane induced changes in nerve conduction velocities and somatosensory evoked potentials. Int. Arch. occup. environ. Health, 51: 45-54.

MUTTI, A., FALZOI, M., LUCERTINI, S., ARFINI, G., ZIGNANI, M., LOMBARDI, S., & FRANCHINI, I. (1984) n-Hexane metabolism in occupationally exposed workers. Br. J. ind. Med., 41: 533-538.

NAKAJIMA, T. & MURAYAMA, N. (1985) Polyneuropathy caused by n-hexane used under the commercial name of "benzine". Ind. Health, 27: 340-341.

NÄSLUND, B.M.A. & HALPERT, J.S. (1984) Selective inhibition by chloramphenicol of cytochrome P-450 isozymes in rat lung and liver involved in the hydroxylation of n-hexane. J. Pharmacol. exp. Ther., 231(1): 16-22.

NELLIGAN, R.E. (1962) Hydrocarbons in the Los Angeles atmosphere. Arch. environ. Health, 5: 581-591.

NELSON, K.W., EGE, J.F., ROSS, M., WOODMAN, L.E., & SILVERMAN, L. (1943) Sensory response to certain industrial solvent vapours. J. ind. Hyg. Toxicol., 25: 282-285.

NICKELSEN, R.L., RODER, M.M., & BERARDINELLI (1986) Permeation of chemical protective clothing by three binary solvent mixtures. Am. Ind. Hyg. Assoc. J., 47: 236-240.

NILSEN, O.G., TOFTGARD, R., ENG, L., & GUSTAFSSON, J. (1981) Regio-specificity of purified forms of rabbit liver microsomal cytochrome P-450 in the metabolism of benzo(a)pyrene, n-hexane and 7-ethoxyresorufin. Acta pharmacol. toxicol., 48: 369-376.

NIOSH (1977a) Criteria for a recommended standard: Occupational exposure to alkanes (C5-C8), Cincinnati, Ohio, National Institute for Occupational Safety and Health (DHEW (NIOSH) Publication No. 77-151).

NIOSH (1977b) NIOSH manual on analytical methods, 2nd ed., Cincinnati, Ohio, National Institute for Occupational Safety and Health, Vol. 1 (DHEW Publication No. (NIOSH) 77-157-A).

NIOSH (1981a) Health hazard evaluation report, Cincinnati, Ohio, National Institute for Occupational Safety and Health (HHE-80-040-860).

NIOSH (1981b) Health hazard evaluation report, Cincinnati, Ohio, National Institute for Occupational Safety and Health (HHE-81-240-1031).

NIOSH (1983) Health hazard evaluation report, Cincinnati, Ohio, National Institute for Occupational Safety and Health (HETA-80-256-1386).

NIOSH (1984) Manual of analytical methods: Hydrocarbons method 1500, Cincinnati, Ohio, National Institute for Occupational Safety and Health, pp. 1500/1-1500/7.

NIOSH (1988) Testimony to DOL on the Occupational Safety and Health Administration's proposed rule on air contaminants, Cincinnati, Ohio, National Institute for Occupational Safety and Health (Pocket No. H-020).

NOLTING, F., BEHNKE, W., & ZETZSCH, C. (1988) A smog chamber for studies of the reactions of terpenes and alkanes with ozone and OH. J. atmos. Chem., 6: 47-59.

NOMEIR, A.A. & ABOU-DONIA, M.B. (1985) Analysis of n-hexane, 2-hexanone, 2,5-hexanedione, and related chemicals by capillary gas chromatography and high-performance liquid chromatography. Anal. Biochem., 151: 381-388.

NOMIYAMA, K. & NOMIYAMA, H. (1974a) Respiratory retention, uptake and excretion of organic solvents in man. Benzene, toluene, n-hexane, trichloro-ethylene, acetone, ethylacetate and ethyl alcohol. Int. Arch. Arbeitsmed., 32: 75-83.

NOMIYAMA, K. & NOMIYAMA, H. (1974b) Respiratory elimination of organic solvents in man. Benzene, toluene, n-hexane, trichloroethylene, acetone, ethylacetate and ethyl alcohol. Int. Arch. Arbeitsmed., 32: 85-91.

NOMIYAMA, K. & NOMIYAMA, H. (1975) [Concerning the cutaneous absorption of n-hexane in humans.] Jpn. J. Hyg., 30: 140 (in Japanese).

NOMIYAMA, K., YOSHIDA, T., & YANAGISAWA, H. (1973) [Percutaneous absorption of n-hexane caused severe polyneuropathy.] In: [Proceedings of the 46th Annual Meeting of the Japanese Association of Industrial Health], Tokyo, Japanese Association of Industrial Health, pp. 560-561 (in Japanese).

NOTTEN, W.R.F. & HENDERSON, P.T. (1975a) The influence of n-hexane treatment on the glucuronic acid pathway and activity of some drug metabolizing enzymes in guinea pig. Biochem. Pharmacol., 24: 127-131.

NOTTEN, W.R.F. & HENDERSON, P.T. (1975b) Action of n-alkanes on drug-metabolizing enzymes from guinea-pig liver. Biochem. Pharmacol., 24: 1093-1097.

NYLEN, P., EBENDAL, T., ERIKSDOTTER-NILSSON, M., HANSSON, T., HENSCHEN, A., JOHNSON, A.C., KRONEVI, T., KVIST, U., SJOSTRAND, N.O., HOGLUND, G., & OLSUN, L. (1989) Testicular atrophy and loss of nerve growth factor - immunoreactive germ cell line in rats exposed to n-hexane and a protective effect of simultaneous exposure to toluene or xylene. Arch. Toxicol., **63**: 296-307.

O'DONOGHUE, J.L. (1985) Alkanes, alcohols, ketones and ethylene oxide. In: O'Donoghue, J.L., ed. Neurotoxicology of industrial and commercial chemicals, Boca Raton, Florida, CRC Press, Vol. 2, pp. 61-97.

O'DONOGHUE, J.L., KRASAVAGE, W.J., & TERHAAR, C.J. (1978a) A comparative chronic toxicity study of methyl n-propyl ketone, methyl n-butyl ketone, and hexane by ingestion, Rochester, New York, Eastman Kodak Company (Unpublished Report No. 104657Y).

O'DONOGHUE, J.L., KRASAVAGE, W.J., & TERHAAR, C.J. (1978b) Toxic effects of 2,5-hexanedione. Toxicol. appl. Pharmacol., **45**: 269 (abstract 115).

OETTEL, H. (1936) [The influence of organic liquids on skin.] Arch. exp. Pathol. Pharmacol., **38**: 641-696 (in German).

OISHI, H. & MINENO, K. (1964) [Polyneuropathy caused by an organic solvent (n-hexane).] Saigai-Igaku, 7(4): 218-222 (in Japanese).

OKAMOTO, S., SHIRBAE, T., KURIMARA, T., & ARAKI, S. (1977) [A case of n-hexane polyneuropathy occurring in an interior decorator and experimental n-hexane neuropathy in rats.] Clin. Neurol. (Tokyo), **17**: 237-242 (in Japanese).

ONO, Y. & TAKEUCHI, Y. (1980) [Polyneuropathy thought to be petroleum benzine poisoning occurring in a worker engaged in cleaning gas meters.] Sangyo Igaku, **22**: 256-262 (in Japanese).

ONO, Y., TAKEUCHI, Y., & HISANAGA, N. (1979) [Studies on the method of measuring nerve conduction velocity in rat's tail and on the comparative toxicity of n-hexane, methyl n-butyl ketone and 2,5-hexanedione.] Jpn. J. ind. Health, **21**: 528-538 (in Japanese with English summary).

ONO, Y., TAKEUCHI, Y., & HISANAGA, N. (1981) A comparative study on the toxicity of n-hexane and its isomers on the peripheral nerve. Int. Arch. occup. environ. Health, **48**: 289-294.

ONO, Y., TAKEUCHI, Y., HISANAGA, N., IWATA, M., KITOH, J., & SUGIURA, Y. (1982) Neurotoxicity of petroleum benzine compared with n-hexane. Int. Arch. occup. environ. Health, **50**: 219-229.

ONOSAKA, S., OCHI, Y., MIN, K.-S., FUJITA, Y., & TANAKA, K. (1988) [Influences of compounds on metallothionein concentration in mouse tissues: II. Decrease of pancreatic metallothionein concentration by n-hexane.] Eisei Kagaku, **34**: 446-450 (in Japanese).

OSHA (Occupational Safety and Health Administration) (1989) Air contaminants: Final rule. Fed. Reg., **54**(12): 2921, 2939 (29 CFR Part 1910).

PALAO, A. & LAJO, J.L. (1981) [Toxic polyneuropathy as a consequence of the use of glue and chemical solvents in the shoe industry.] Arch. Neurobiol., **44**(1): 35-48 (in Spanish).

PARLATO, G., INSERRA, A., & TIMPANARO, V. (1968) Electrocardiographic changes in experimental poisoning with liquid hydrocarbons (petrol ether, hexane and heptane). Folia med., 51: 799-805.

PASTERNAK, T., FLOOD, D.G., ESKIN, T.A., & MERIGAN, W.H. (1985). Selective damage to large cells in the cat retinogeniculate pathway by 2,5-hexanedione. J. Neurosci., 5: 1641-1652.

PATTY, F.A. & YANT, W.P. (1929) Odour intensity and symptoms produced by commercial propane, butane, pentane, hexane and heptane vapour, Washington, DC, US Bureau of Mines, 10 pp (Report No. RI 2979).

PAULSON, G.W. & WAYLONIS, G.W. (1976) Polyneuropathy due to n-hexane. Arch. intern. Med., 136: 880-882.

PELLIN, M.C., VILANOVA, E., & BARRIL, J. (1988) Low non-neuropathic tri-o-cresyl phosphate (TOCP) doses inhibit neuropathy target esterase near the neuropathic threshold in n-hexane pretreated hens. Toxicology, 49: 99-105.

PELLIZZARI, E.D., HARTWELL, T.D., HARRIS, B.S.H., WADDELL, R.D., WHITAKER, D.A., & ERICKSON, M.D. (1982) Purgeable organic compounds in mother's milk. Bull. environ. Contamin. Toxicol., 28: 322-328.

PERBELLINI, L. & BRUGNONE, F. (1980) Identification of the metabolites of n-hexane, cyclohexane and their isomers in men's urine. Toxicol. appl. Pharmacol., 53: 220-229.

PERBELLINI, L., BRUGNONE, F., PASTORELLO, G., & GRIGOLINI, L. (1979) Urinary excretion of n-hexane metabolites in rats and humans. Int. Arch. occup. environ. Health, 42: 349-354.

PERBELLINI, L., BRUGNONE, F., & GAFFURI, E. (1981a) Neurotoxic metabolites of "commercial hexane" in the urine of shoe factory workers. Clin. Toxicol., 18(12): 1377-1385.

PERBELLINI, L., BRUGNONE, F., & FAGGIONATO, G. (1981b) Urinary excretion of the metabolites of n-hexane and its isomers during occupational exposure. Br. J. ind. Med., 38: 20-26.

PERBELLINI, L., BRUGNONE, F., SILVESTRI, R., & GAFFURI, E. (1981c) Measurement of the urinary metabolites of n-hexane, cyclohexane and their isomers by gas chromatography. Int. Arch. occup. environ. Health, 48: 99-106.

PERBELLINI, L., BRUGNONE, F., & GAFFURI, E. (1981d) [Occupational health hazard of technical hexane: study of the biotransformation products extracted from urine.] Ann. Ist. Sup. Sanità., 17: 615-620 (in Italian).

PERBELLINI, L., AMANTINI, M.C., BRUGNONE, F., & FRONTALI, N. (1982a) Urinary excretion of n-hexane metabolites. A comparative study in rat, rabbit and monkey. Arch. Toxicol., 50: 203-215.

PERBELLINI, L., LEONE, R., FRACASSO, M.E., BRUGNONE, F., & VENTURINI, M.S. (1982b) Metabolic interaction between n-hexane and toluene *in vivo* and *in vitro*. Int. Arch. occup. environ. Health, 50: 351-358.

PERBELLINI, L., BARTOLUCCI, G.B. BRUGNONE, F., DE ROSA, E., & VALENTINI, F. (1985a) [2,5-Hexanedione in the biological monitoring of occupational exposure to n-hexane.] Med. Lav., 76(1): 35-43 (in Italian).

PERBELLINI, L., BRUGNONE, F., CARETTA, D., & MARANELLI, G. (1985b) Partition coefficients of some industrial aliphatic hydrocarbons (C5-C7) in blood and human tissues. Br. J. ind. Med., 42: 162-167.

PERBELLINI, L., BRUGNONE, F., MOZZO, P., DE ROSA, E., BARTOLUCCI, B., & FACINNI, G. (1985c) Toxicokinetic aspects of n-hexane 2,5-hexanedione in the biomonitoring of occupational exposure to n-hexane. Annu. Conf. Ind. Hyg., 12: 357-364.

PERBELLINI, L., MOZZO, P., BRUGNONE, F., & ZEDDE, A. (1986) Physiologico-mathematical model for studying human exposure to organic solvents: kinetics of blood/tissue n-hexane concentrations and of 2,5-hexanedione in urine. Br. J. ind. Med., 43: 760-768.

PEROCCO, P., BOLOGNESI, S., & ALBERGHINI, W. (1983) Toxic activity of seventeen industrial solvents and halogenated compounds on human lymphocytes cultured in vitro. Toxicol. Lett., 16: 69-75.

PETERS, M.A., HUDSON, P.M., & DIXON, R.L. (1981) The effect of totigestational exposure to methyl n-butyl ketone has on postnatal development and behaviour. Ecotoxicol. environ. Saf., 5: 291-306.

PLANAS, A.M. & CUNNINGHAM, V.J. (1987) Uncoupling of cerebral glucose supply and utilization after hexane-2,5-dione intoxication in the rat. J. Neurochem., 48: 816-823.

PRYOR, G.T. & HOWD, R.A. (1982) Developmental long-term effects of inhalants in animals, Washington, DC, National Institute of Drug Abuse (NIDA Quarterly Report No. 5).

PRYOR, G.T., BINGHAM, J., DICKINSON, J., REBERT, C.S., & HOWD, R.A. (1982) Importance of schedule of exposure to hexane in causing neurotoxicity. Neurobehav. Toxicol. Teratol., 4: 71-78.

PRYOR, G.T., DICKINSON, J., HOWD, R.A., & REBERT, C.S. (1983) Neuro-behavioural effects of subchronic exposure of weanling rats to toluene or hexane. Neurobehav. Toxicol. Teratol., 5: 47-52.

RABOVSKY, J. & JUDY, D.J. (1989) The *in vitro* effects of alkanes, alcohols, and ketones on rat lung cytochrome P450-dependent alkoxyphenoxazone dealkylase activities. Arch. Toxicol., 63: 13-17.

RABOVSKY, J., JUDY, D.J., & PAILES, W.H. (1986) *In vitro* effects of straight-chain alkanes (n-hexane through n-dodecane) on rat liver and lung cytochrome P.450. J. Toxicol. environ. Health, 18: 409-421.

RAITTA, C., SEPPALAINEN, A.M., & HUUSKONEN, M.S. (1978) n-Hexane maculopathy in industrial workers. Albrecht Graefes Arch. klin. exp. Ophthalmol., 209: 99-110.

RAJE, R.R. (1983) *In vitro* toxicity of n-hexane and 2,5-hexanedione using isolated perfused rabbit heart. J. Toxicol. environ. Health, 11: 879-884.

RAJE, R.R., GREENING, M., & FINE, M.T. (1984) Blood n-hexane concentration following acute inhalation exposure in rats. Res. Commun. chem. Pathol. Pharmacol., 46(2): 297-300.

RALSTON, W.H., HILDERBRAND, R.L., UDDIN, D.E., ANDERSEN, M.E., & GARDINER, R.W. (1985) Potentiation of 2,5-hexanedione neurotoxicity by methyl ethyl ketone. Toxicol. appl. Pharmacol., 81: 319-327.

RANADIVE, K.J., GOTHOSKAR, S.V., & TEZABWALA, B.U. (1972) Carcinogenicity of contaminants in indigenous edible oils. Int. J. Cancer, 10: 652-666.

RAPPAPORT, S.M., SELVIN, S., & WATERS, M.A. (1987) Exposures to hydrocarbon components of gasoline in the petroleum industry. Appl. ind. Hyg., 2: 148-154.

REBERT, C.S. & SORENSON, S.S. (1983) Concentration-related effects of hexane on evoked responses from brain and peripheral nerve of the rat. Neurobehav. Toxicol. Teratol., 5: 69-76.

REBERT, C.S., HOUGHTON, P.W., HOWD, R.A., & PRYOR, G.T. (1982) Effects of hexane on the brainstem auditory response and caudal nerve action potential. Neurobehav. Toxicol. Teratol., 4: 79-85.

RIZZUTO, N., TERZIAN, H., & GALIAZZO-RIZZUTO, S. (1977) Toxic polyneuropathies in Italy due to leather cement poisoning in the shoe industries. A light and electron microscope study. J. neurol. Sci., 31: 343-354.

RIZZUTO, N., DECRANDIS, D., DITRAPANI, G., & PASTINATO, E. (1980) n-Hexane neuropathy. An occupational disease of shoemakers. Eur. Neurol., 19(5): 308-315.

ROBERTSON, P., WHITE, E.L., & BUS, J.S. (1982) Effect of methyl ethyl ketone treatment on hepatic mixed function oxidase activity and on in vivo metabolism of n-hexane. Toxicologist, 2(2): A273.

ROBERTSON, P., Jr, WHITE, E.L., & BUS, J.S. (1989) Effects of methyl ethyl ketone pretreatment on hepatic mixed function oxidase activity and on *in vivo* metabolism of n-hexane. Xenobiotica, 19: 721-729.

ROSENBERG, C.K., ANTHONY, D.C., SZAKAL-QUIN, G., GENTER, M.B., & GRAHAM, D.G. (1987a) Hyperbaric oxygen accelerates the neurotoxicity of 2,5-hexanedione. Toxicol. appl. Pharmacol., 87: 374-379.

ROSENBERG, C.K., GENTER, M.B., SZAKAL-QUIN, G., ANTHONY, D.C., & GRAHAM, D.G. (1987b) dl-versus meso-3,4-dimethyl-2,5-hexanedione: a morphometric study of the proximo-distal distribution of axonal swellings in the anterior root of the rat. Toxicol. appl. Pharmacol., 87: 363-373.

RUFF, R.L., PETITO, C.K., & ACHESON, L.S. (1981) Neuropathy associated with chronic low level exposure to n-hexane. Clin. Toxicol., 18(5): 515-519.

SABRI, M. (1984) *In vitro* effects of n-hexane and its metabolites on selected enzymes in glycolysis, pentose phosphate pathway and citric acid cycle. Brain Res., **297**: 145-150.

SABRI, M., MOORE, C.L., & SPENCER, P.S. (1979) Studies on the biochemical basis of distal axonopathies. I. Inhibition of glycolysis by neurotoxic hexacarbon compounds. J. Neurochem., **32**: 683-689.

SAHU, S.C., LOWTHER, D.E., & JONES, S.L. (1982) Biochemical response of rat lung to inhaled n-hexane. Toxicol. Lett., **12**: 13-17.

SAIDA, K., MENDELL, J.R., & WEISS, H.S. (1976) Peripheral nerve changes induced by methyl n-butyl ketone and potentiation by methyl ethyl ketone. J. Neuropathol. exp. Neurol., **35**(3): 207-225.

SANAGI, S., SEKI, Y., SUGIMOTO, K., & HIRATA, M. (1980) Peripheral nervous system functions of workers exposed to n-hexane at a low level. Int. Arch. occup. environ. Health, **47**: 69-79.

SANDMEYER, E.E. (1981) Aliphatic hydrocarbons. In: Clayton, G.D. & Clayton, F.E., ed. Patty's industrial hygiene and toxicology, 3rd ed., New York, Chichester, Brisbane, Toronto, John Wiley and Sons, Vol. 2B, pp. 3175-3220.

SAX, N.I. (1984) Dangerous properties of industrial materials, 6th ed., New York, Van Nostrand Reinhold Company.

SAYRE, L.M., SHEARSON, C.M., WONGMONGKOLRIT, T., MEDORI, R., & GAMBETTI, P. (1986) Structural basis of c-diketone neurotoxicity: non-neurotoxicity of 3,3-dimethyl-2,5-hexanedione, a c-diketone incapable of pyrolle formation. Toxicol. appl. Pharmacol., **84**: 36-44.

SCELSI, R., POGGI, P., FERA, L., & GONELLA, G. (1980) Toxic polyneuropathy due to n-hexane. J. neurol. Sci., **47**: 7-19.

SCELSI, R., POGGI, P., FERA, L., & GONELLA, G. (1981) Industrial neuropathy due to n-hexane and 2,5-hexanedione. Clinical and morphological findings in three cases. Clin. Toxicol., **18**: 1387-1393.

SCHAUMBURG, H.H. & SPENCER, P.S. (1976) Degeneration in central and peripheral nervous systems produced by pure n-hexane: an experimental study. Brain, **99**: 183-192.

SCHAUMBURG, H.H. & SPENCER, P.S. (1979) Clinical and experimental studies of distal axonopathy. A frequent form of brain and nerve damage produced by environmental chemical hazards. Ann. NY Acad. Sci., **329**: 14-29.

SCHNOY, N., SCHMIDT, R., ALTENKIRCH, H., & WAGNER, H.M. (1982) Ultrastructural alteration of alveolar epithelium after exposure to organic solvents. Respiration, **43**: 221-231.

SCHMIDT, R., SCHNOY, N., ALTENKIRCH, H., & WAGNER, H.M. (1984) Ultrastructural alteration of intrapulmonary nerves after exposure to organic solvents. Respiration, **46**: 362-369.

SELKOE, D.J., LUCKENBILL-EDDS, L., & SHELANSKI, M.L. (1978) Effects of neurotoxic industrial solvents on cultured neuroblastoma cells: methyl n-methyl ketone, n-hexane and derivatives. J. Neuropathol. exp. Neurol., 37: 768-789.

SEPPALAINEN, A. & RAITTA, C. (1981) Neurotoxic properties of n-hexane among occupationally exposed workers. In: Proceedings of the 2nd Finnish-Estonian Symposium on Early Effects of Toxic Substances, Helsinki, June 1981, Helsinki, Institute of Occupational Health, pp. 180-184.

SEPPALAINEN, A., RAITTA, C., & HUUSKONEN, M. (1979) n-Hexane induced changes in visual evoked potentials and electroretinograms of industrial workers. Electroencephalogr. clin. Neurophysiol., 47: 492-498.

SHIRBAE, T., TSUDA, T., TERAO, A., & ARAKI, S. (1974) Toxic polyneuropathy due to glue sniffing. J. neurol. Sci., 21: 101-113.

SICE, J. (1966) Tumour-promoting activity of n-alkanes and 1-alkanols. Toxicol. appl. Pharmacol., 9: 70-74.

SINGH, D. & JAIN, D.C. (1987) Relative toxicity of various organic solvents generally used in screening plant products for insecticidal activity against the house fly *Musca domestica L.* Indian J. exp. Biol., 25: 569-570.

SINGH, K.P., KANNAN, K., GOEL, S.K., PANDYA, K.P., & SHANKER, R. (1983) 2,5-Hexanediol induced thymic atrophy and lymphocytotoxicity in rats. Ind. Health, 21: 235-242.

SINGH, K.P., UPRETI, R.K., SAXENA, A.K., & SHANKER, R. (1984) Thymic toxicity produced by 2,5-hexanediol and 2,5-hexanedione in rats. In: Proceedings of the International Conference on Organic Solvents Toxicity, Stockholm, October 1984, p. 144 (Abstract 550).

SOBUE, I. & YAMAMURA, Y. (1968) [n-Hexane polyneuropathy. Outbreak among vinyl sandal manufacturers.] Rinsho Shinkei, 8: 393-403 (in Japanese).

SOBUE, I., IIDA, M., YAMAMURA, Y., & TAKAYANAGUI, T. (1978) n-Hexane polyneuropathy. Int. J. Neurol., 11(4): 317-330.

SPAGNA, C., PARLATO, G., & TIMPANARO, V. (1967) [Behaviour of blood picture in experimental hexane intoxication.] Folia med. (Napoli), 50: 977-985 (in Italian).

SPENCER, P. (1981) Morphological study of n-hexane intoxication: Final report, Washington, DC, American Petroleum Institute (Attachment to API Medical Research Publication No. 28-30077).

SPENCER, P. (1982) Neuropathic potential of n-hexane in the presence of other hexane isomers, Washington, DC, American Petroleum Institute (API Medical Research Publication No. 30-30226).

SPENCER, P.S. & SCHAUMBURG, H.H. (1977a) Ultrastructural studies of the dying-back process. III. The evolution of experimental peripheral giant axonal degeneration. J. Neuropathol. exp. Neurol., 36: 276-299.

SPENCER, P.S. & SCHAUMBURG, H.H. (1977b) Ultrastructural studies of the dying-back process. IV. Differential vulnerability of PNS and CNS fibres in experimental central-peripheral distal axonopathies. J. Neuropathol. exp. Neurol., 36: 300-320.

SPENCER, P.S., SCHAUMBURG, H.H., SABRI, M.I., & VERONES, B. (1980) The enlarging view of hexacarbon neurotoxicity. CRC crit. Rev. Toxicol., 17(4): 279-356.

STOLTENBURG-DIDINGER, G., WAGNER, H.M., & ALTENKIRCH, H. (1984) Embryo and fetotoxicity of n-hexane and methyl ethyl ketone. In: Proceedings of the International Conference on Organic Solvent Toxicity, Stockholm, October 1984, p. 125 (Abstract 405).

STRATTON, G.W. & SMITH, T.M. (1988) Interaction of organic solvents with the green alga *Chlorella pyrenoidosa*. Bull. environ. Contam. Toxicol., 40: 736-742.

SUZUKI, T., SHIMBO, S., & NISHITANI, H. (1974) Muscular atrophy due to glue sniffing. Int. Arch. Arbeitsmed., 33: 115-123.

SVABOVA, E., ZORAD, S., MITKOVA, A., KLIMES, I., & MACHO, L. (1987) [Increase of insulin binding and degradation on isolated human erythrocytes by n-heptane and n-hexane; effects of trypsin and dithiotreitol.] Bratisl. lek. Listy., 88(6): 615-624 (in Slovak).

SWANN, H.E., KWON, B.K., HOGAN, G.K., & SNELLINGS, W.M. (1974) Acute inhalation toxicology of volatile hydrocarbons. Am. Ind. Hyg. Assoc. J., 35: 511-518.

TAIRA, M. (1975) [Experimental studies on pathomorphological changes of lung produced by aliphatic and aromatic hydrocarbons and gasoline.] J. Tokyo med. Univ., 33(4): 597-607 (in Japanese).

TAKAHASHI, M., TAKEUCHI, H., KYO, S., YORIFUJI, S., SANAGI, SL., SEKI, Y., & HARA, I. (1977) n-Hexane polyneuropathy: a case report with review of literature. Med. J. Osaka Univ., 28(1): 77-85.

TAKEUCHI, Y., MABUCHI, C., & TAKAGI, S. (1975) Polyneuropathy caused by petroleum benzine. Int. Arch. Arbeitsmed., 34: 185-197.

TAKEUCHI, Y., ONO, Y., HISANAGA, N., KITOH, J., & SUGIURA, Y. (1980) A comparative study on the neurotoxicity of n-pentane, n-hexane and n-heptane in the rat. Br. J. ind. Med., 37: 241-247.

TAKEUCHI, Y., ONO, Y., & HISANAGA, N. (1981) An experimental study on the combined effects of n-hexane and toluene on the peripheral nerve of the rat. Br. J. ind. Med., 38: 14-19.

TAKEUCHI, Y., ONO, Y., HISANAGA, N., IWATA, M., AOYAMA, M., KITOH, J., & SUGIURA, Y. (1983) An experimental study of the combined effects of n-hexane and methyl ethyl ketone. Br. J. ind. Med., 40: 199-203.

THAM, R., BUNNFORS, I., ERIKSSON, B., LARSBY, B., LINDGREN, S., & ODKVIST. L. (1984) Vestibulo-ocular disturbances in rats exposed to organic solvents. Acta pharmacol. toxicol., 54: 58-63.

TIL, H.P., FALKE, H.E., BEEMS, R.B., BRUIJNTJES, J.P., & DE VOGEL, N. (1989) Subchronic (90-day) oral toxicity study in rats, including metaphase chromosomal analysis of bone marrow cells, with light petroleum solvent (technical hexane) for oil seed extraction: Final report, Zeist, The Netherlands, TNO-CIVO Institutes, 166 pp (Project No. B/88-0541) (Report No. V/89.089).

TOFTGARD, R., NILSEN, O.G., & GUSTAFSSON, J.A. (1981) Changes in rat liver microsomal cytochrome P-450 and enzymatic activities after the inhalation of n-hexane, xylene, methyl ethyl ketone and methyl chloroform for four weeks. Scand. J. Work Environ. Health, 7: 31-37.

TOFTGARD, R., NILSEN, O.G., GLAUMANN, H., & GUSTAFSSON, J.A. (1983) Induction of cytochrome P-450 in the rat liver after exposure to xylenes. Dose response relationship and dependence on endocrine factors. Toxicology, 27: 119-137.

TOFTGARD, R., HAAPARANTA, T., ENG, L., & HALPERT, J. (1984) Rat lung and liver microsomal cytochrome P-450 isozymes involved in the hydroxylation of n-hexane and m-xylene. In: Abstracts of the International Conference on Organic Solvent Toxicity, Stockholm, October 1984, p. 17 (Abstract 111).

TOFTGARD, R., HAAPARANTA, T., ENG, L., & HALPERT, J. (1986) Rat lung and liver microsomal cytochrome P-450 isozymes involved in the hydroxylation of n-hexane. Biochem. Pharmacol., 35: 3733-3738.

TOWFIGHI, J., NICHOLAS, K., GONATAS, M.D., PLEASURE, D., COOPER, H.S., & MCCREE, L. (1976) Glue sniffer's neuropathy. Neurology, 26: 238-243.

TOXIGENICS (1982) 90-Day vapour inhalation toxicity study on n-hexane in albino rats (Report submitted to Chemical Industry Institute of Toxicology, North Carolina) (CIIT Pocket No. 10242).

TSURUTA, H. (1977) Percutaneous absorption of organic solvents. II. A method for measuring the penetration rate of chlorinated solvents through excised rat skin. Ind. Health, 15: 131-139.

TSURUTA, H. (1980) Microdetermination of n-hexane in biological samples by gas chromatography - mass spectroscopy. Ind. Health, 18: 113-114.

TSURUTA, H. (1982) Percutaneous absorption of organic solvents. III. On the penetration rates of hydrophobic solvents through the excised rat skin. Ind. Health, 20: 335-345.

UPRETI, R.K., SINGH, K.P., SAXENA, A.K., & SHANKER, R. (1986) Effect of 2,5-hexanedione on lymphoid organs in rats: a preliminary report. Environ. Res., 39: 188-198.

USITC (1988) Synthetic organic chemicals. United States Production and Sales 1987, Washington, DC, United States International Trade Commission, pp. 2-7 (USITC Publication No. 2009).

VAINIO, H. (1974) Activation and inactivation of membrane-bound UDP-glucuronosyltransferase by organic solvents *in vitro*. Acta pharmacol. toxicol., **34**: 152-156.

VDI (Verband Deutscher Ingenieure) (1984) Handbook of clean air, Berlin, Benth Verlag Gmbh, Vol. 5 (Guideline 3482).

VERONESI, B., PETERSON, E.R., DI VINCENCO, G., & SPENCER, P.S. (1978) A tissue culture model of distal (dying-back) axonopathy: its use in determining primary neurotoxic hexacarbon compounds. J. Neuropathol. exp. Neurol., **33**: 703.

VERONESI, B., PETERSON, E.R., & SPENCER, P.S. (1980) Reproduction and analysis of MnBK neurotoxicity in organotypic tissue culture. In: Spencer, P.S. & Schaumburg, H.H., ed. Experimental and clinical neurotoxicology, Baltimore, Maryland, Williams and Wilkins, pp. 863-871.

VERONESI, B., PETERSON, E.R., BORNSTEIN, M., & SPENCER, P.S. (1983) Ultrastructural studies of the dying-back process. VI. Examination of nerve fibres undergoing giant axonal degeneration in organotypic culture. J. Neuropathol. exp. Neurol., **42**(2): 153-165.

VERONESI, B., LINGTON, A.W., & SPENCER, P.S. (1984) A tissue culture model of methyl ethyl ketone's potentiation of n-hexane neurotoxicity. Neurotoxicology, **5**(2): 43-52.

VEULEMANS, H., VAN VLEM, E., JANSSENS, H., MASSCHELEIN, R., & LEPLAT, A. (1982) Experimental human exposure to n-hexane. Study of the respiratory uptake and elimination, and of n-hexane concentrations in peripheral venous blood. Int. Arch. occup. environ. Health, **49**: 251-263.

VEULEMANS, H., GROESENEKEN, D., MASSCHELEIN, R., & VLEM, E.V. (1987) Survey of ethylene glycol ether exposures in Belgian industries and workshops. Am. Ind. Hyg. Assoc. J., **48**: 671-676.

VICEDO, J.L., PELLIN, M., & VILLANOVA, E. (1985) Phthalates and organo-phosphorus compounds as cholinesterase inhibitors in fractions of industrial hexane impurities. Arch. Toxicol., **57**: 46-52.

VILANOVA, E. & VICEDO, J.L. (1983) Serum cholinesterase inhibitors in the commercial hexane impurities. Arch. Toxicol., **53**: 59-69.

WADA, Y., OKAMOTO, S., & TAKAGI, S. (1965) [Intoxication polyneuropathy following exposure to n-hexane.] Rinsho Shinkeigaku, **10**(5): 591-597 (in Japanese).

WAGNER, H.M., STEPPART, R., & ALTENKIRCH, H. (1984) [Animal experiments on the neurotoxicity of organic solvents in rats challenged with heavy metals.] Schriftenr. Ver. Wasser Boden Lufthyg., **59**: 191-200 (in German).

WAHLBERG, J.E. (1984a) Erythema-inducing effects of solvents following epicutaneous administration to man: studied by laser Doppler flowmetry. Scand. J. Work Environ. Health, **10**: 159-162.

WAHLBERG, J.E. (1984b) Edema inducing effects of solvents following topical administration. Derm. Beruf Umwelt, **32**(3): 91-94.

WAHLBERG, J.E. & BOMAN, A. (1979) Comparative percutaneous toxicity of ten industrial solvents in the guinea-pig. Scand. J. Work Environ. Health, **5**: 345-351.

WALSETH, F. & NILSEN, O.G. (1984) Phthalate esters. II. Effects of inhaled dibutylphthalate on cytochrome P-450 mediated metabolism in rat liver and lung. Arch. Toxicol., **55**: 132-136.

WALSETH, F., TOFTGARD, R., & NILSEN, O.G. (1982) Phthalate esters. I. Effects on cytochrome P-450 mediated metabolism in rat liver and lung, serum enzymatic activities and serum protein levels. Arch. Toxicol., **50**: 1-10.

WANG, J.D., CHANG, Y.C., KAO, K.P., HUANG, C.C., LIN, C.C., & YEH, W.Y. (1986) An outbreak of n-hexane induced polyneuropathy among press proofing workers in Taipei. Am. J. ind. Med., **10**: 111-118.

WEAST, R.C. (1981) CRC handbook of chemistry and physics, 6th ed., Boca Raton, Florida, CRC Press.

WHITE, E.L. & BUS, J.S. (1980) Determination of n-hexane, methyl ethyl ketone and their metabolites in sciatic nerves of rats by gas chromatography-mass spectrometry. In: Abstracts of the Pittsburgh Conference on Analytical Chemistry and Applied Spectroscopy, 10-14 March, 1980, Pittsburgh, Pennsylvania, US Society of Analytical Chemistry (Abstract No. 525).

WHITE, E.L., BUS, J.S., & HECK, H. (1979) Simultaneous determination of n-hexane, 2-hexanone and 2,5-hexanedione in biological tissues by gas chromatography mass spectrometry. Biomed. mass Spectrom. **6**(4): 169-172.

WHO (1971) Evaluation of food additives. Fourteenth Report of the Joint FAO/WHO Expert Committee on Food Additives, Geneva, World Health Organization, pp. 21-24 (Technical Report Series No. 462).

YAMADA, N. (1964) [Polyneuritis in workers handling n-hexane.] Sangyo Igaku, **6**: 192 (in Japanese).

YAMADA, S. (1967) [Intoxication polyneuritis in workers exposed to n-hexane.] Jpn. J. ind. Health, **9**: 651-659 (in Japanese).

YAMAKAGE, A. & ISHIKAWA, H. (1982) Generalised morphea-like scleroderma occurring in people exposed to organic solvents. Dermatologia, **165**: 186-193.

YAMAMURA, Y. (1969) n-Hexane polyneuropathy. Folia psychiatr. neurol. Jpn.,23(1): 45-57.

YOSHIDA, T., YANAGISAWA, H., MUNEYUKI, T., & SHIGIYA, R. (1974) [An electrophysiological study of n-hexane polyneuropathy.] Rinsho Shinkeigaku, 14(5): 454-461 (in Japanese).

ZAHLSEN, K., AARSTAD, K., & NILSEN, O.G. (1985) Inhalation of isopropanol. Induction of activating and deactivating enzymes in rat kidney and liver. Increased microsomal metabolism of n-hexane. Toxicology, 34: 57-66.

RESUME

Le *n*-hexane (hexane normal) est un liquide volatil incolore. L'hexane du commerce se présente essentiellement sous la forme d'un mélange de divers isomères de l'hexane et de dérivés apparentés à six atomes de carbone; sa teneur en *n*-hexane varie entre 20 et 80%. La chromatographie en phase gazeuse avec détection par ionisation de flamme ou couplage à un spectrographe de masse constitue une bonne technique pour le dosage du *n*-hexane. Les limites d'exposition professionnelle varient de 100 à 1800 mg/m^3 (moyenne pondérée par rapport au temps, TWA) et de 400 à 1500 mg/m^3 (valeur plafond, CLV) selon les pays.

On peut isoler le *n*-hexane du gaz naturel et du pétrole brut. On l'utilise dans les industries de transformation alimentaire, notamment pour l'extraction des huiles végétales ou comme solvant dans différents produits et procédés.

Une fois libéré dans l'environnement, le *n*-hexane y subsiste essentiellement en phase vapeur. Sa demi-vie dans l'atmosphère est estimée à environ deux jours, si l'on se base uniquement sur sa réactivité vis-à-vis du radical OH. Les valeurs de la CL$_{50}$ pour les organismes aquatiques sont rares et dispersées; elles ont été obtenues dans des conditions peu satisfaisantes. Dans ces conditions il n'est pas possible d'apprécier les effets toxiques du *n*-hexane dans l'environnement. Du fait de sa faible solubilité dans l'eau et de sa forte volatilité il est peu probable que les organismes aquatiques courent un risque d'exposition, sauf en cas de décharge sauvage dans les eaux superficielles.

Chez les mammifères, le *n*-hexane est rapidement résorbé au niveau des poumons et se distribue largement dans l'organisme de l'adulte ainsi que dans les tissus du foetus. Au niveau cutané, la résorption est faible. Le *n*-hexane subit une métabolisation oxydative en un certain nombre de dérivés, notamment l'hexane-2,5-dione dont on pense qu'elle constitue l'agent neurotoxique final. Dans le nerf sciatique de rats d'expérience on a pu trouver des concentrations particulièrement élevées de *n*-hexane et d'hexane-2,5-dione. La majeure partie du *n*-hexane est excrétée sans modification dans l'air exhalé; une certaine quantité est également excrétée sous forme de métabolites dans l'air expiré et dans les urines.

Le *n*-hexane présente une faible toxicité aiguë pour le rat adulte après administration par voie orale ou inhalation. On a noté des valeurs de la DL_{50} par voie orale allant de 15 à 30 g/kg; quant à la CL_{50} par inhalation, elle serait de 271 040 mg/m³ (77 000 ppm) pour une exposition d'une heure. Lorsque la teneur en vapeurs est élevée, on constate chez l'animal de l'ataxie, des convulsions et les signes d'une dépression du système nerveux central.

Il semble que chez le rat, les principaux effets d'une exposition répétée au *n*-hexane consistent en lésions testiculaires et signes de neurotoxicité. C'est ainsi que l'inhalation de *n*-hexane et l'ingestion d'hexane-2,5-dione ont produit de graves lésions testiculaires chez les animaux d'expérience. Ces effets ont été attribués à la désagrégation du cytosquelette des cellules de Sertoli. On note des effets secondaires sur les cellules germinales des stades postérieurs aux spermatogonies, qui disparaissent des tubules endommagés. Après une seule exposition de 24 heures à 17 600 mg/m³ de *n*-hexane (5000 ppm) les effets testiculaires étaient réversibles mais ils devenaient irréversibles après deux semaines d'exposition à la même concentration, 16 heures par jour, six jours par semaine. A la concentration de 1% dans l'eau de boisson, l'hexane-2,5-dione a produit des lésions testiculaires réversibles du même type au bout de deux à trois semaines d'administration et des effets irréversibles (en l'espace de 17 semaines) au bout de cinq semaines d'administration.

L'effet neurotoxique se caractérise cliniquement par une faiblesse des pattes arrières qui peut évoluer vers la paralysie. Il se produit un gonflement de l'axone aux niveaux central et périphérique avec parfois des lésions plus sévères (dégénérescence et disparition de l'axone), notamment au niveau des troncs nerveux de plus grande longueur et de plus gros diamètre. Lors d'études comportant principalement l'inhalation d'hexane pendant six mois, on a noté la présence de lésions du système nerveux central et périphérique aux doses de 1760 mg/m³ (500 ppm) ou davantage; en revanche il n'y avait pas d'effets cliniques ou anatomopathologiques à la dose de 400 mg/m³ (125 ppm). Quinze à 22 semaines après l'arrêt de l'exposition, cinq jours par semaine pendant 11 semaines à des vapeurs de *n*-hexane à la concentration de 3520 mg/m³ (1000 ppm), on a noté que l'amplitude des potentiels évoqués auditifs du tronc cérébral (PEAP) n'était que partiellement restaurée. L'exposition discontinue de rats à une concentration de 3168 mg/m³ (900 ppm) pendant 72 semaines n'a pas provoqué de lésions apparentes aux niveaux périphérique ou central mais certains effets électrophysiologiques étaient perceptibles au niveau des nerfs périphériques.

La neurotoxicité induite par le *n*-hexane peut être potentialisée en présence de méthyléthylcétone, de méthylisobutylcétone et d'acétate de plomb et réduite par exposition simultanée au toluène. La perturbation des concentrations de dopamine est également synergisée par une exposition simultanée au toluène et au *n*-hexane.

Des lésions microscopiques graves ont été observées sur la peau après application de *n*-hexane et pose d'un pansement occlusif après une brève période. L'exposition prolongée à des vapeurs de *n*-hexane à une concentration de 1560 mg/m³ (3000 ppm) peut provoquer chez le rat une irritation des conjonctives et une forte irritation oculaire chez le lapin. On ne dispose d'aucune donnée sur la sensibilisation cutanée provenant d'études sur l'animal.

Des lésions chromosomiques (polyploïdie dans le cas d'une étude, et aberrations de structure dans le cas d'une autre) ont été signalées tant *in vitro* qu'*in vivo*. On n'a pas observé d'augmentation de la fréquence des mutations ponctuelles ni de signes de lésion de l'ADN.

Une étude de cancérogénicité a été effectuée sur des souris (badigeonnage de la peau avec du *n*-hexane): elle n'a révélé aucun signe de cancérogénicité.

Les effets du *n*-hexane sur la fonction de reproduction n'ont pas été suffisamment étudiés. Aucun signe important d'embryotoxicité ou de tératogénicité n'a été observé chez des rats après inhalation de *n*-hexane à des concentrations relativement basses ni chez des souris après administration par voie orale. On a constaté un retard transitoire du développement postnatal chez des ratons après exposition des femelles gravides à des vapeurs de *n*-hexane à des concentrations de 3520 mg/m³ (1000 ppm).

On ne possède guère de données sur la toxicité aiguë du *n*-hexane pour l'être humain. La plupart des études portent sur l'exposition professionnelle à des mélanges de solvants. D'après les données disponibles, il semble que le *n*-hexane n'ait qu'une faible toxicité aiguë. On a signalé des signes de dépression du système nerveux central, tels que somnolence, vertiges, sensation ébrieuse, après exposition à de l'hexane du commerce pendant 10 à 60 minutes à des concentrations allant de 3520 à 17 600 mg/m³ (1000-5000 ppm).

Le *n*-hexane est légèrement irritant et provoque un érythème passager chez l'homme après un court contact cutané. Des effets plus graves (érythème et phlyctènes) ont été enregistrés après un contact de cinq heures avec du *n*-hexane de qualité commerciale, la zone de contact étant recouverte. Aucun cas de sensibilisation cutanée n'a été signalé chez les ouvriers exposés et un test de sensibilisation cutanée maximale effectué avec du *n*-hexane a donné des résultats négatifs.

En cas d'exposition répétée, le *n*-hexane entraîne une polynévrite sensitivo-motrice périphérique. De nombreuses études sur la prévalence des effets neurotoxiques dus au *n*-hexane ont été publiées; toutefois on manque bien souvent de données satisfaisantes sur l'exposition. Des cas de neuropathie ont été attribués à l'exposition à des concentrations atmosphériques de *n*-hexane allant de 106 à 8800 mg/m³ (30-2500 ppm). Des cas de neuropathie périphérique marquée ont été signalés parmi des ouvriers japonais travaillant à la fabrication de sandales ainsi que chez des opérateurs taïwanais de presse à épreuves exposés à des teneurs en *n*-hexane d'environ 76 et 352 mg/m³ (50 et 100 ppm), respectivement, pendant des périodes supérieures à huit heures par jour. Dans la plupart des cas, les mesures d'exposition étaient récentes et ne reflétaient probablement pas très exactement les expositions antérieures susceptibles d'être à l'origine de la neuropathie en question.

Plusieurs études transversales ont fait état, indépendamment les unes des autres, d'effets infracliniques légers (par exemple des altérations électrophysiologiques au niveau des nerfs périphériques) chez des travailleurs exposés à des concentrations de 70-352 mg/m^3 (20-100 ppm). Aucun cas bien défini de neurophathie périphérique cliniquement manifeste n'a pu être relevé dans l'une quelconque de ces études à des niveaux d'exposition inférieurs à 352 mg/m^3 (100 ppm).

Seuls quelques travaux ont été consacrés à l'étude des effets du *n*-hexane sur le système nerveux central. On pense que les modifications observées dans les potentiels évoqués somatosensoriels d'ouvriers exposés à du *n*-hexane proviennent d'un bloc de la conduction nerveuse centrale. On a également noté une altération des potentiels évoqués visuels et du tracé électro-encéphalographique. Ces résultats incitent à penser que le *n*-hexane pourrait entraîner des troubles du système nerveux central, mais les données disponibles ne donnent aucune indication sur les niveaux d'exposition en cause.

EVALUATION DES RISQUES POUR LA SANTE HUMAINE ET DES EFFETS SUR L'ENVIRONNEMENT

1. Etudes sur l'animal

1.1 Exposition à court et à long terme

Le n-hexane présente une faible toxicité aiguë puisque l'on fait état de valeurs de la DL_{50} comprises entre 15 et 30 g/kg et d'une valeur de la CL_{50} à une heure de 271 040 mg.

Lors d'études consistant essentiellement à faire inhaler du n-hexane à des rats de manière continue, on a observé une mortalité chez ces animaux après exposition à une concentration de 3520 mg/m^3 (1000 ppm) pendant des durées allant jusqu'à 11 semaines, ainsi qu'une diminution du gain de poids après trois semaines d'exposition à 1760 mg/m^3 (500 ppm). Lors d'études comportant des expositions quotidiennes de 12 heures à du n-hexane, on a enregistré une mortalité chez les animaux à la concentration de 10 560 mg/m^3 (3000 ppm) au bout de 15 semaines et une légère réduction du gain de poids corporel à la concentration de 740 mg/m^3 (200 ppm) au bout de 24 semaines. Aucun effet sur le poids corporel des rats n'a été observé après une exposition pratiquement continue à 443 mg/m^3 (126 ppm) pendant 34 semaines.

Il semble que les lésions testiculaires et les effets neurotoxiques aux niveaux périphérique et central soient les principaux effets non mortels d'une exposition répétée au n-hexane chez le rat. Après inhalation de n-hexane et ingestion de hexane-2,5-dione on a observé de graves lésions testiculaires. Ces effets ont été attribués à la désagrégation du cytosquelette des cellules de Sertoli. On observe également des effets secondaires sur les cellules germinales des stades qui suivent la spermatogonie et qui disparaissent des tubules endommagés. Après une seule exposition de 24 heures à 17 600 mg/m^3 (5000 ppm), les effets testiculaires étaient réversibles mais ils devenaient irréversibles après deux semaines d'exposition à la même concentration 16 heures par jour, six jours par semaine. De l'hexane-2,5-dione administrée dans l'eau de boisson à la concentration de 1% a produit des lésions testiculaires réversibles au bout de deux à trois semaines d'administration et des effets irréversibles (en l'espace de 17 semaines) au bout de cinq semaines d'administration.

Du point de vue clinique, la neurotoxicité se caractérise par une faiblesse des pattes arrières, qui peut évoluer vers la paralysie et aboutir à une quadriplégie. Ces signes cliniques ont été observés après dix semaines d'exposition discontinue à 10 560 mg/m^3 (3000 ppm) (12 heures par jour et sept jours par semaine) et au bout de six à dix semaines d'exposition continue à des doses allant de 1048-2112 mg/m^3 (400 à 600 ppm).

Avant que ne se manifeste la faiblesse des pattes arrières on a observé des lésions (gonflement de l'axone) au niveau des nerfs des pattes arrières, du cerveau et de la moëlle épinière. Des effets plus graves (dégénérescence et disparition de l'axone) ont été notés en particulier au niveau des troncs nerveux de plus grande longueur et plus grand diamètre au bout de six mois d'exposition à 1760 mg/m^3 (500 ppm). Au total, il est difficile d'établir la valeur de la dose sans effet nocif observable dans le cas des effets neurotoxiques provoqués par le *n*-hexane chez le rat, en raison de la diversité des concentrations et des modalités d'exposition expérimentées ainsi que de la variété des effets étudiés. Lors d'études de six mois consistant essentiellement à faire inhaler en continu des vapeurs de *n*-hexane, on a observé des lésions nerveuses à des concentrations de 1760 mg/m^3 (500 ppm ou davantage), toutefois aucun effet clinique ni anatomopathologique n'a été constaté à la dose de 440 mg/m^3 (125 ppm). En mode discontinu l'exposition de rats à la dose de 3168 mg/m^3 (900 ppm) pendant 72 semaines n'a pas provoqué de lésions nerveuses évidentes, mais on a pu constater les premiers signes d'effets sur la force de préhension.

Après arrêt de l'exposition il peut y avoir résolution (partielle ou complète) des signes cliniques de toxicité, de l'amoindrissement de la force de préhension et des effets électrophysiologiques. Dans les 15 à 22 semaines qui suivent l'arrêt d'une exposition répétée à la concentration de 3520 mg/m^3 (1000 pmm) de *n*-hexane pendant 11 semaines, on constate que l'amplitude de l'onde cinq des potentiels évoqués auditifs du tronc cérébral (qui est supposée refléter l'activité du système nerveux central) ainsi que le potentiel d'action du nerf caudal, ne sont pas complètement rétablis. On n'a pas encore étudié systématiquement la résolution des lésions anatomopathologiques consécutives à une exposition par inhalation, mais on a toutefois observé que lorsqu'on cesse d'exposer les animaux à des concentrations allant de 1408 à 2112 mg/m^3 (400 à 600 ppm), il y a remyélinisation et régénération limitées des axones.

L'inhalation en discontinu pendant sept semaines de *n*-hexane à la concentration de 1760 mg/m^3 (500 ppm) peut provoquer de petites lésions au niveau des poumons chez le rat. Chez le lapin, on a observé de graves lésions de l'arbre respiratoire après exposition à une concentration de 10 560 mg/m^3 (3000 ppm), huit heures par jour pendant huit jours, et on a noté une prolifération papillaire des cellules broncholiaires non ciliées au bout de 24 semaines d'exposition.

On a fait état d'effets sur le rein et le foie à la suite de quelques études d'inhalation sur des rats mais seulement aux doses les plus fortes. Quant à la plupart des autres lésions et des autres effets, on a estimé qu'ils étaient d'une importance toxicologique mineure ou constaté qu'ils n'étaient pas reproductibles. Cependant, on a observé de graves lésions hépatiques chez des rats après administration intrapéritonéale répétée de *n*-hexane.

Des études portant sur l'exposition à plusieurs solvants ont montré que les effets neurotoxiques de la vapeur de *n*-hexane pouvaient être accrus chez des poules par la présence de méthyl-isobutylcétone et chez des rats par la présence simultanée de méthyl-isobutylcétone et d'acétate de plomb; toutefois l'effet était au contraire réduit en présence de toluène. On a également indiqué que les lésions pulmonaires observées chez les rats augmentaient en cas d'exposition simultanée à la méthyléthylcétone et à l'hexane.

Peu d'études ont été consacrées aux effets de l'ingestion de *n*-hexane ou à ceux de l'exposition cutanée à cette substance. L'administration quotidienne par voie orale de 500 mg/kg de *n*-hexane pendant quatre semaines à des rats a entraîné une baisse de la vitesse de conduction du nerf caudal.

1.2 Génotoxicité

Le *n*-hexane a fait l'objet de tests de mutagénicité limités. On a fait état de lésions chromosomiques (polyploïdie dans le cas d'une étude et aberrations structurales dans le cas d'une autre) lors d'essais *in vitro* au cours desquels une lignée cellulaire provenant de hamsters chinois a été exposée à du *n*-hexane liquide non dilué en l'absence de fraction métabolisante. Dans le cas de cellules mammaliennes en culture ou de bactéries, on n'a pas observé d'augmentation significative du taux de mutations ponctuelles. L'exposition au *n*-hexane n'augmente pas les lésions de l'ADN comme on a pu en juger par des mesures de toxicité bactérienne différentielle. De même il n'y a pas d'augmentation de la synthèse non programmée d'ADN dans les lymphocytes humains *in vitro*. Bien que les tests portant sur les mutations ponctuelles aient donné des résultats négatifs, il semble, à certains signes, que le *n*-hexane soit capable de produire des aberrations chromosomiques *in vitro*. Des lésions chromosomiques (rupture des chromatides) ont été signalées à l'occasion d'une étude *in vivo* sur des cellules de moëlle osseuse de rat.

1.3 Cancérogénicité

Le pouvoir cancérogène du *n*-hexane n'a pas été suffisamment étudié. Une étude de portée limitée a montré que l'application cutanée de *n*-hexane ne semblait pas accroître la formation de tumeurs cutanées chez la souris après exposition à un initiateur tumoral (diméthyl-7,12 benzanthracène) ou après exposition simultanée à un agent promoteur (huile de croton).

1.4 Effets sur la reproduction

Les effets toxiques du *n*-hexane sur la fonction de reproduction n'ont pas été convenablement étudiés. Il n'existe pas de preuves substantielles que le *n*-hexane entraîne des effets embryotoxiques ou tératogènes après inhalation chez le rat ou ingestion chez la souris. Chez des rats exposés à une dose de 10 560 mg/m^3 (3000 ppm), on a observé une légère augmentation de l'incidence de certaines anomalies, toutefois en raison d'insuffisances dans la manière dont l'étude a été conduite (par exemple concentration probablement trop faible) les conclusions qu'on peut en tirer demeurent limitées. Des signes de toxicité foetale (réduction du poids des souriceaux) ont été observés mais seulement à des doses qui entraînaient une mortalité importante chez les femelles gravides. Une des études effectuées a mis en évidence un retard passager dans le développement postnatal de ratons exposés à la concentration de 10 560 mg/m^3 (3000 ppm). Aucun signe de neuropathie n'a été signalé chez ces animaux mais on n'est pas en mesure, sur la base des résultats de cette étude, de se prononcer sur la possibilité que l'exposition *in utero* au *n*-hexane induise effectivement une neuropathie, car les animaux n'ont été exposés à cette substance que durant une courte fraction de la période de gestation. Selon d'autres rapports, l'exposition *in utero* au *n*-hexane retarderait la genèse du tissu cérébelleux ainsi que la maturation des neurones et produirait des anomalies électrophysiologiques au niveau central chez les rats nouveaux-nés. Cependant on ne possède pas suffisamment de détails sur ces travaux pour en apprécier toute la portée.

On est fondé à penser que le *n*-hexane entraîne une stérilité irréversible chez le rat. Une étude limitée de dominance létale chez la souris n'a pas révélé d'effets sur la fertilité des mâles. Aucune étude n'a été publiée sur la fertilité des femelles de divers animaux ou sur les effets portant sur plusieurs générations.

2. Etudes sur l'homme

2.1 Effets sur le système nerveux

Selon de nombreuses études un certain nombre de cas humains de neuropathie périphérique seraient imputables à une exposition professionnelle au *n*-hexane. Toutefois les concentrations atmosphériques sont rarement mentionnées et quand elles le sont, elles peuvent très bien être inexactes, sans compter qu'il n'est pas toujours facile de savoir s'il s'agit d'hexane ou de *n*-hexane. En outre, l'exposition au *n*-hexane en milieu industriel se produit généralement lors de l'utilisation de produits contenant divers solvants, de sorte que les ouvriers sont exposés en fait à un mélange de composés volatils (par exemple de l'acétate d'éthyle, de la méthyléthylcétone, du toluène, de l'acétone et des hydrocarbures aliphatiques autres que le *n*-hexane). La concentration atmosphérique des autres solvants présents est rarement précisée. Dans la présente mise au point, on ne prend en considération que celles des études qui donnent les concentrations atmosphériques.

Les résultats de l'étude électrophysiologique des nerfs périphériques peuvent varier considérablement selon la technique utilisée, la température du laboratoire dans lequel les mesures sont effectuées, la portion du nerf étudiée et l'âge du sujet. Aussi est-il difficile d'apprécier la portée des études qui reposent sur ces méthodes, en l'absence de renseignements sur tous ces facteurs.

L'étude de 93 cas de neuropathie a permis de caractériser le tableau clinique de la neuropathie due au *n*-hexane et a montré que les données électrophysiologiques étaient en bonne corrélation avec la gravité de la maladie. On a en particulier constaté que plus l'exposition était importante plus la maladie était grave. Toutefois il n'a pas été possible d'établir une relation bien définie à partir des données limitées dont on disposait sur l'exposition effective.

On a observé de légers signes infracliniques de neuropathie chez des ouvriers d'une fabrique de chaussures exposés à une concentration de 70 mg/m^3 (20 ppm). L'importance des anomalies électrophysiologiques augmentait avec la durée de l'exposition. Toutefois aucun cas de neuropathie déclarée n'a été observé même chez les ouvriers qui avaient été exposés pendant plus de cinq ans.

On a observé des signes subjectifs et électrophysiologiques de neuropathie périphérique infraclinique dans un groupe d'ouvriers exposés à une dose d'environ 317 mg/m^3 (90 ppm). Toutefois, on ne peut pas attribuer entièrement ces effets à l'exposition au *n*-hexane étant donné que l'on a probablement sous-estimé les expositions antérieures à divers solvants et que les ouvriers avaient probablement introduit eux-mêmes un biais sélectif. En outre, il peut y avoir eu exposition simultanée à de la méthyléthylcétone, dont on sait qu'elle accroît les effets neurotoxiques du *n*-hexane.

L'exposition à un mélange de solvants contenant du *n*-hexane à la concentration d'environ 690 mg/m³ (196 ppm) a entraîné une réduction de la vitesse de conduction nerveuse périphérique, anomalie qui s'est maintenue même après une réduction importante de l'exposition. En outre, on pense que les variations observées dans les potentiels évoqués somatosensoriels s'expliquent par l'effet du *n*-hexane sur le système nerveux central.

Des signes subjectifs et électrophysiologiques d'une neuropathie infraclinique légère ont été observés dans un petit groupe de travailleurs exposés à une concentration moyenne de *n*-hexane dans l'atmosphère de 208 mg/m³ (59 ppm). Aucun signe clinique de neuropathie n'était perceptible. L'exposition à d'autres solvants était limitée et on a pu procéder à des études de conduction nerveuse dans des conditions bien définies. Toutefois, le faible effectif des ouvriers, l'absence de données rétrospectives sur l'exposition et le fait que les groupes témoins n'étaient pas très bien appariés au groupe exposé limitent la portée des conclusions qu'on peut en tirer. Néanmoins, les résultats sont en bon accord général avec les données fournies par les études antérieures dont il a été question plus haut. On a attribué le déclenchement d'une neuropathie périphérique cliniquement manifeste à l'exposition pendant des périodes supérieures à huit heures par jour à une concentration de *n*-hexane de 669 mg/m³ (190 ppm). Au bout d'un certain nombre d'années, on assiste à une lente restauration - encore que partielle - de la fonction nerveuse. L'exposition à une concentration inférieure à 352 mg/m³ (100 ppm) n'a pas entraîné de neuropathie mais l'étude électrophysiologique a révélé la présence d'effets infracliniques.

Chez un petit nombre de travailleurs exposés de par leur profession à toute une gamme de concentrations atmosphériques de *n*-hexane, on a observé une perturbation de la perception des couleurs et des signes de maculopathie. La mesure des potentiels évoqués visuels et l'électrorétinogramme ont révélé chez ces sujets la présence d'anomalies par comparaison avec un groupe témoin non exposé. On a également signalé l'existence d'anomalies dans les potentiels évoqués visuels chez des renifleurs de colle exposés à du *n*-hexane. On pense qu'il pourrait se produire une dégénérescence axonale au niveau des voies optiques et un bloc de conduction au niveau central. On est également fondé à croire que les signes de maculopathie pourraient être corrélés avec les signes électrophysiologiques de neuropathie périphérique. Certains des sujets étudiés présentaient également un électroencéphalogramme anormal.

2.2 Autres effets

Aucune étude n'a été publiée au sujet d'effets éventuels sur les testicules et la fertilité des mâles. On ne dispose que de très peu d'informations sur la toxicité aiguë du *n*-hexane pour l'homme. La plupart des études toxicologiques portaient sur l'exposition à des mélanges de solvants.

A la lumière des données disponibles, il semble que le *n*-hexane n'ait qu'une faible toxicité aiguë.

Très peu d'études portant sur des volontaires ont été publiées à propos du pouvoir irritant de *n*-hexane pour la peau et les yeux. Le *n*-hexane est légèrement irritant et il provoque l'apparition d'un érythème passager après un bref contact avec la peau. Des effets plus graves (érythème et formation de phlyctènes) ont été observés après un contact cutané de cinq heures avec de l'hexane de qualité commerciale, la zone touchée étant recouverte. On n'a pas suffisamment de données pour se prononcer sur le pouvoir irritant de l'hexane liquide pour l'oeil humain. Lors d'une étude au cours de laquelle des volontaires ont été exposés à de la vapeur d'hexane à une concentration de 1760 mg/m^3 (500 ppm) pendant trois à cinq minutes, on a relevé aucun signe d'irritation oculaire. Il n'a pas non plus été fait état de sensibilisation cutanée chez des ouvriers exposés, ni lors d'un test de sensibilisation maximale effectué avec ce produit.

3. Effets sur l'environnement

Le *n*-hexane est peu soluble dans l'eau et extrêmement volatil. Les organismes aquatiques sont donc peu exposés à cette substance; une exposition passagère peut cependant se produire en cas de décharge sauvage dans les eaux superficielles. Les données dont on dispose sur la toxicité du *n*-hexane pour les organismes aquatiques sont très peu nombreuses; elles sont très diverses et ont été obtenues dans des conditions peu satisfaisantes; dans ces conditions, elles ne permettent pas d'évaluer convenablement le risque pour l'environnement.

RECOMMANDATIONS

1. Protection de la santé humaine

Les concentrations de n-hexane auxquelles la population est exposée dans son ensemble, ne représentent pour elle aucun danger. Dans les ambiances de travail, il convient de maintenir les teneurs dans l'atmosphère endessous des limites recommandées pour l'exposition professionnelle en recourant à des procédés convenablement étudiés et en utilisant certains dispositifs mécaniques, notamment la ventilation. Dans les milieux confinés, en cas d'urgence et lors de certaines opérations d'entretien, il est souhaitable que des vêtements spéciaux et une protection respiratoire appropriée soient mis à la disposition du personnel. Il est recommandé d'utiliser un appareil respiratoire autonome à débit continu pour des concentrations de n-hexane allant jusqu'à 8800 mg par m³ (2500 ppm). Entre 880mg/m³ (2550 ppm) et 17 600 mg/m³ (5000 ppm), l'appareil respiratoire doit comporter un masque facial complet. Les gants protecteurs résistent, semble-t-il, à la pénétration du n-hexane mais certains mélanges de n-hexane avec d'autres solvants tels que la méthyléthylcétone pourraient faciliter la pénétration du n-hexane à travers le tissu des gants ou des vêtements protecteurs. C'est un facteur à prendre en compte lorsqu'on utilise du n-hexane en mélange avec d'autres solvants.

2. Protection de l'environnement

Il est peu probable que le n-hexane présente un danger pour l'environnement, sauf en cas de décharge ou de déversement très importants, auquel cas des effets passagers peuvent se produire.

RECHERCHES A EFFECTUER

a) Il faudrait étudier la fonction testiculaire au moyen d'un certain nombre d'indices parmi des groupes de travailleurs exposés de par leur profession, afin d'établir si l'un ou la totalité des effets observés chez l'animal se produisent également chez l'homme.

b) Il conviendrait d'étudier plus à fond *in vivo* les effets génotoxiques du *n*-hexane afin de compléter les données limitées obtenues *in vitro*.

c) Il est nécessaire de procéder à une étude comportant une exposition répétée au *n*-hexane afin d'établir quelle est sa toxicité par voie orale. C'est à partir des résultats obtenus qu'on pourra déterminer la dose sans effet nocif observable qui permettra de fixer une DJA.

d) Le mécanisme de la neurotoxicité reste obscur au niveau moléculaire. L'élucidation de ce mécanisme est d'un intérêt direct en vue d'une estimation valable du risque encouru. Des études *in vivo* et *in vitro* sont nécessaires pour étudier plus à fond et clarifier ces mécanismes.

d) Les études de tératogénicité existantes ne permettent pas d'évaluer le risque. D'autres études sont à entreprendre pour que l'on puisse disposer de données utilisables.

f) On n'a pas pu établir de relations dose-réponse nettes en ce qui concerne les effets neurotoxiques du *n*-hexane chez l'homme car les données relatives à l'exposition sont soit incomplètes soit peu fiables. En outre, même si l'on a amplement démontré l'existence d'effets neurotoxiques périphériques, les effets sur le système nerveux central n'ont pas été suffisamment étudiés. Il importe d'entreprendre d'autres études épidémiologiques, notamment des études longitudinales prospectives, afin de combler les lacunes des travaux antérieurs.

RESUMEN

El *n*-hexano (hexano normal) es un líquido volátil e incoloro. El hexano comercial está formado principalmente por una mezcla de isómeros del hexano y de compuestos afines de seis átomos de carbono; su contenido de *n*-hexano oscila entre el 20 y el 80%. Un sistema adecuado para la medida del *n*-hexano es la combinación de la cromatografía de gases con la detección de ionización por conductor o la espectroscopía de masa. Los límites de la exposición profesional varían entre 100-1800 mg/m^3 (promedio ponderado en el tiempo) y 400-1500 mg/m^3 (valor máximo) en diversos países.

El *n*-hexano se puede aislar del gas natural y del petróleo crudo. Se utiliza en la elaboración de alimentos, inclusive en la extracción de aceite vegetal, y como disolvente en varios productos y procesos.

Una vez liberado en el medio ambiente, el *n*-hexano se encuentra fundamentalmente en fase de vapor. Se estima que su semivida en la atmósfera es de unos 2 días, de acuerdo con su reactividad con el radical OH solo. Los valores descritos de la CL_{50} para los organismos acuáticos son pocos y variables, y se han determinado en condiciones inadecuadas; por consiguiente, no es posible valorar los efectos tóxicos del *n*-hexano en el medio ambiente. Su baja solubilidad en agua y su elevada volatilidad hacen improbable la exposición de los organismos acuáticos, salvo en el caso de vertido incontrolado en aguas de superficie.

En los mamíferos, el *n*-hexano se absorbe rápidamente a través de los pulmones y se distribuye por todo el cuerpo adulto, así como en los tejidos fetales. La absorción cutánea es limitada. El *n*-hexano sufre un metabolismo oxidativo y da diversos compuestos, entre los que se encuentra la 2,5-hexanodiona, considerada el agente neurotóxico final. En el nervio ciático de las ratas se pueden encontrar niveles particularmente elevados de *n*-hexano y de 2,5-hexanodiona. La mayor parte del *n*-hexano se elimina inalterado en el aire exhalado; otra parte se excreta metabolizado en el aire exhalado y la orina.

El n-hexano administrado a ratas adultas por vía oral o respiratoria tiene una toxicidad aguda baja. Para una hora de exposición se han registrado valores de DL_{50} de 15-30 g/kg por vía oral y de 271 040 mg/m^3 (77 000 ppm) por vía respiratoria. En concentraciones altas de vapor, los animales muestran ataxia, convulsiones y signos de depresión del sistema nervioso central.

Parece ser que el efecto principal de la exposición repetida al n-hexano en ratas es la aparición de lesiones testiculares y neurotoxicidad. La exposición por vía respiratoria al n-hexano y por vía oral a la 2,5-hexanodiona produjeron lesiones testiculares graves. Estos efectos se han atribuido a la alteración del citoesqueleto de las células de Sertoli. Se producen efectos secundarios en las células germinales postespermatogónicas, que desaparecen de los túbulos afectados. Los efectos testiculares fueron reversibles tras la exposición única durante 24 h a 17 600 mg/m^3 (5000 ppm) pero irreversibles tras exposiciones de 16 h/día y 6 días/semana durante dos semanas a la misma concentración. La ingestión de agua de bebida con un 1% de 2,5-hexanodiona durante dos o tres semanas produjo lesiones testiculares reversibles análogas y efectos irreversibles (en un plazo de 17 semanas) tras cinco semanas de tratamiento.

El efecto neurotóxico se caracteriza clínicamente por debilidad en las extremidades posteriores, que puede llegar a la parálisis. En el sistema nervioso central y periférico se produce inflamación axonal; se pueden presentar lesiones más graves (degeneración y pérdida axonal) sobre todo en los nervios más largos y de diámetro mayor. En estudios de inhalación prácticamente continua durante seis meses con dosis de 1760 mg/m^3 (500 ppm) o superiores se produjeron lesiones en el sistema nervioso periférico y central, pero no se observaron efectos clínicos o patológicos a concentraciones de 440 mg/m^3 (125 ppm). De 15 a 22 semanas después de cesar la exposición constante a una concentración de vapor de 3520 mg por m^3 (1000 ppm), cinco días a la semana durante 11 semanas, sólo se había producido una recuperación limitada de la amplitud de la respuesta evocada por un estímulo auditivo del quinto par craneal (que se considera que indica actividad del sistema nervioso central) y del potencial de acción del nervio de la cola. La exposición discontinua de ratas a una concentración de 3168 mg/m³ (900 ppm) durante 72 semanas no causó ninguna lesión evidente en el sistema nervioso periférico o central, pero se observaron indicios de efectos electrofisiológicos en los nervios periféricos.

La neurotoxicidad inducida por el *n*-hexano puede aumentar con la exposición simultánea a metiletilcetona, metilisobutilcetona y acetato de plomo y disminuir con la exposición simultánea al tolueno. El tolueno y el *n*-hexano ejercen también un efecto sinérgico en la alteración de los niveles de dopamina.

Tras la aplicación cutánea de *n*-hexano en condiciones oclusivas durante períodos cortos se observó en la piel la aparición de lesiones microscópicas graves. La exposición prolongada a una concentración de vapor de *n*-hexano de 10 560 mg/m³ (3000 ppm) puede ocasionar irritación de la conjuntiva en la rata y pronunciada irritación ocular en el conejo. No se dispone de datos sobre sensibilización cutánea a partir de estudios en animales.

Se ha informado de la aparición de lesiones cromosómicas (poliploidía en un estudio y aberraciones estructurales en otro) en experimentos tanto *in vivo* como *in vitro*. En las pruebas realizadas para determinar las lesiones en el ADN no se ha observado aumento de la frecuencia de las mutaciones puntuales ni de los efectos en ellas.

Se ha realizado un estudio de la carcinogenicidad del *n*-hexano (pintando la piel de ratones), que resultó negativo.

No se ha estudiado lo bastante la toxicidad del *n*-hexano para la reproducción. No se observaron indicios claros de que su inhalación tenga en las ratas efectos embriotóxicos o teratogénicos, aunque las concentraciones utilizadas fueron relativamente bajas, y tampoco en ratones después de la administración oral. Cuando, en un estudio con ratas, se expusieron a las madres a una concentración de vapor de *n*-hexano de 3520 mg/m³ (1000 ppm), se retrasó de forma pasajera el desarrollo postnatal de la descendencia.

Se dispone de muy poca información acerca de la toxicidad aguda del *n*-hexano en la especie humana. La mayor parte de los estudios se han centrado en la exposición profesional a mezclas de disolventes. Los datos disponibles indican que el n-hexano tiene una toxicidad aguda escasa. Se han señalado manifestaciones de depresión del sistema nervioso central, como somnolencia, vértigo y mareos, tras la exposición a n-hexano comercial en concentraciones que van de 3520 a 17 600 mg/m^3 (1000-5000 ppm) durante 10-60 minutos.

El n-hexano es una sustancia ligeramente irritante que al entrar en contacto con la piel del hombre durante períodos cortos produce un eritema pasajero. Se ha informado de efectos más graves (eritema y vesículas) tras un contacto cutáneo oclusivo de cinco horas con un hexano de tipo comercial. No se han notificado casos de sensibilización cutánea en trabajadores expuestos, y tampoco se observó en un ensayo de maximización con n-hexano.

Con exposiciones repetidas, el n-hexano es neurotóxico e induce un tipo de neuropatía periférica sensomotora. Se han publicado muchos estudios sobre la prevalencia de la neurotoxicidad inducida por el n-hexano; sin embargo, a menudo se carece de datos adecuados sobre la exposición. La exposición a concentraciones de n-hexano en el aire que oscilan entre 106 y 8800 mg/m^3 (30-2500 ppm) se ha relacionado con neuropatías. Se han descrito casos de acusada neuropatía periférica entre trabajadores japoneses de la industria de las sandalias y en tipógrafos de Taiwán expuestos a niveles de n-hexano de unos 176 y 352 mg/m^3 (50 y 100 ppm), respectivamente, durante períodos superiores a 8 h diarias. En muchos casos las mediciones de la exposición eran recientes y no reflejaban de manera exacta las exposiciones anteriores causantes de neuropatía.

En varios estudios cruzados se han observado por separado efectos subclínicos ligeros (por ejemplo, cambios electrofisiológicos en los nervios periféricos) en trabajadores expuestos a 70-352 mg/m^3 (20-100 ppm). En ninguno de esos estudios se identificaron casos clínicamente evidentes de neuropatía periférica con niveles de exposición inferiores a 352 mg/m^3 (100 ppm).

Sólo en un pequeño número de estudios se han investigado los efectos del n-hexano en el sistema nervioso central. Se ha indicado que los cambios del potencial inducido por estímulos somatosensoriales en trabajadores expuestos al *n*-hexano podrían deberse a un bloqueo de la conducción del sistema nervioso central. También se ha observado una alteración del potencial inducido por estímulos visuales, así como modificaciones electroencefalográficas. Estos resultados parecen indicar que el *n*-hexano puede producir una disfunción del sistema nervioso central. Sin embargo, los datos disponibles no aportan información relativa a los niveles de exposición correspondientes.

EVALUACION DE LOS RIESGOS PARA LA SALUD HUMANA Y DE LOS EFECTOS EN EL MEDIO AMBIENTE

1. Estudios en animales

1.1 Exposición a corto y largo plazo

El *n*-hexano tiene una toxicidad aguda baja; se han comunicado valores de DL_{50} del orden de 15-30 g/kg y una CL_{50} (1 hora) de 271 040 mg/m^3.

En los estudios de inhalación prácticamente continua en ratas se produjo la muerte tras una exposición a 3520 mg/m^3 (1000 ppm) de *n*-hexano durante un período máximo de 11 semanas y se redujo la ganancia de peso corporal después de tres semanas de exposición a 1760 mg/m^3 (500 ppm). En estudios con una exposición diaria de 12 horas al *n*-hexano, se produjo la muerte con una concentración de 10 560 mg/m^3 (3000 ppm) al cabro de 15 semanas, y una ligera disminución de la ganancia de peso corporal con 740 mg/m^3 (200 ppm) después de 24 semanas. No se observaron efectos en el peso corporal en ratas expuestas a 443 mg/m^3 (126 ppm) de manera prácticamente continua durante 34 semanas.

Los principales efectos no letales de la exposición repetida de ratas al *n*-hexano parecen ser la toxicidad testicular y la neurotoxicidad, tanto periférica como central. La exposición respiratoria al *n*-hexano y la oral a la 2,5-hexanodiona producen lesiones testiculares graves. Los efectos se han atribuido a la alteración del citoesqueleto de las células de Sertoli. Hay efectos secundarios en las células germinales postespermatogónicas, que desaparecen de los túbulos afectados. Los efectos testiculares fueron reversibles tras una exposición única de 24 horas a 17 600 mg/m^3 (5000 ppm), pero se hacían irreversibles después de dos semanas de exposición a la misma concentración durante 16 horas/día y 6 días/semana. El agua de bebida con un 1% de 2,5-hexanodiona produjo lesiones testiculares reversibles después de 2-3 semanas de administración, y efectos irreversibles (en un plazo de 17 semanas) tras 5 semanas de tratamiento.

Clínicamente, la neurotoxicidad se caracteriza por debilidad en las extremidades posteriores, que puede evolucioner hasta parálisis y por último tetraplejía. Se han observado manifestaciones clínicas tras 10 semanas de exposición discontinua a 10 560 mg/m^3 (3000 ppm) (12 horas/día, 7 días/semana) y después de 6-10 semanas de exposición continua a una concentración de 1408-2112 mg/m^3 (400-600 ppm).

Antes de la aparición de debilidad en las extremidades posteriores, se observaron lesiones (inflamación axonal) en los nervios de dichas extremidades, en el cerebro y en la médula espinal. Tras seis meses de exposición a 1760 mg/m^3 (500 ppm) se apreciaron efectos más graves (degeneración y pérdida axonal), principalmente en los nervios más largos y de diámetro mayor. En conjunto, resulta difícil determinar el nivel de no observación de efectos adversos correspondiente a la neurotoxicidad inducida por el *n*-hexano en ratas, a causa de la variedad de concentraciones de vapor y de tipos de exposición en las pruebas, y de la diversidad de efectos investigados. En estudios de exposición por inhalación prácticamente continua durante seis meses, se observaron lesiones nerviosas con concentraciones de *n*-hexano de 1760 mg por m^3 (500 ppm) o más, pero no se manifestaron efectos clínicos o patológicos a 440 mg/m^3 (125 ppm). La exposición discontinua de ratas a una concentración de 3168 mg/m^3 (900 ppm) durante 72 semanas no causó ninguna lesión nerviosa manifiesta, pero hubo indicios preliminares de un efecto en la fuerza prensil.

Cuando se interrumpe la exposición pueden desaparecer (parcial o totalmente) los signos clínicos de toxicidad, la disminución de la fuerza prensil y los efectos electrofisiológicos. De 15 a 22 semanas después de cesar la exposición repetida durante 11 semanas a una concentración de 3520 mg/m^3 (1000 ppm), sólo se observó una recuperación limitada de la amplitud de la respuesta inducida por los estímulos auditivos en el quinto componente del tronco encefálico (que se considera que refleja la actividad del sistema nervioso central) y del potencial de acción del nervio caudal. No se ha investigado la desaparición de las lesiones patológicas después de la exposición por vía respiratoria, pero se ha observado remielinización y regeneración axonal limitada al interrumpirse la exposición a concentraciónes de 1408 a 2112 mg/m³ (400-600 ppm).

El tratamiento discontinuo durante siete semanas por vía respiratoria con 1760 mg/m³ (500 ppm) puede causar ligeras lesiones pulmonares en la rata. En conejos se apreciaron, tras la exposición a 10 560 mg/m³ (3000 ppm) 8 horas/día durante 8 días, lesiones graves en el tracto respiratorio y, después de 24 semanas de exposición, proliferaciones papilares de células bronquiolares no ciliadas.

En algunos estudios de inhalación en ratas se han señalado efectos en el riñón y el hígado, pero solo con niveles de exposición más elevados. La mayor parte de las lesiones y otros efectos se consideraron de escasa importancia toxicológica y/o no se reprodujeron en estudios repetidos. Sin embargo, tras la administración intraperitoneal repetida de *n*-hexano a ratas se han observado lesiones hepáticas graves.

Los estudios de exposición combinada han puesto de manifiesto que los efectos neurotóxicos del vapor de *n*-hexano en las gallinas pueden aumentar con la presencia de metilisobutilcetona y en las ratas con la de metilisobutilcetona y acetato de plomo, mientras que el tolueno los hace disminuir. También se ha señalado que la exposición de ratas a la combinación con metiletilcetona aumenta las lesiones pulmonares.

Se han realizado algunos estudios sobre los efectos de la exposición oral o cutánea al *n*-hexano. La administración diaria por vía oral de 500 mg/kg durante cuatro semanas produjo en las ratas una disminución de la velocidad de conducción en el nervio caudal.

1.2 Genotoxicidad

Se han realizado pocas pruebas de mutagenicidad. Se ha informado de la aparición de lesiones cromosómicas (poliploidía en un estudio, y aberraciones estructurales en otro) en ensayos *in vitro*, en los que se expuso una línea celular de hámster chino a *n*-hexano líquido no diluido en ausencia de fracción metabolizante. Tras la exposición de células cultivadas de mamíferos o de bacterias a *n*-hexano no se produjo un aumento significativo del índice de mutaciones puntuales. Las lesiones en el ADN, medidas en ensayos de toxicidad diferencial en bacterias, no aumentaron por la exposición al *n*-hexano. Tampoco observó aumento de la síntesis no programada del ADN en linfocitos humanos *in vitro*. Aunque el *n*-hexano ha dado resultados negativos en los ensayos para detectar mutaciones puntuales, hay algunas pruebas de que puede producir aberraciones cromosómicas *in vitro*. En un estudio *in vivo* con células de médula ósea de rata se informó de lesiones cromosómicas (roturas cromatídicas).

1.3 Carcinogenicidad

No se ha estudiado de manera adecuada el potencial carcinogénico del *n*-hexano. En un estudio limitado de aplicación en la piel a ratones, no pareció que aumentase la formación de tumores cutáneos tras la exposición a un iniciador cancerígeno (7,12-dimetilbenzantraceno) o junto con un agente promotor (aceite de crotón).

1.4 Efectos en la reproducción

No se ha investigado debidamente la toxicidad del *n*-hexano para la reproducción. No hay pruebas sólidas de embriotoxicidad o teratogenicidad en las ratas tras su inhalación, ni tampoco en los ratones después de la administración oral. En ratas expuestas a una concentración de 10 560 mg/m^3 (3000 ppm) se observó un ligero aumento de la incidencia de algunas anomalías, pero las deficiencias de método del estudio (por ejemplo, es probable que las concentraciones ensayadas no fueran lo bastante altas) limita el valor de las conclusiones. En ratones se detectaron signos de fetotoxicidad (menor peso de las crías), pero sólo con dosis que provocaron una letalidad considerable en las madres. En un estudio con crías de ratas expuestas a una concentración de 10 560 mg/m^3 (3000 ppm) se informó de un retraso pasajero del desarrollo postnatal. Aunque no se describieron signos de neuropatía en esos animales, no es posible evaluar a partir de ese estudio si la podría inducir la exposición *in utero*, puesto que los animales sólo estuvieron expuestos al *n*-hexano durante una pequeña parte del período de gestación. En otros informes se ha afirmado que la exposición *in utero* al *n*-hexano retarda la histogénesis cerebelar y la maduración neuronal e induce anomalías electrofisiológicas en el sistema nervioso central de ratas recién nacidas. Sin embargo, este trabajo no se ha expuesto con suficiente detalle para hacer una evaluación completa.

Existen pruebas de que el *n*-hexano causa esterilidad irreversible en las ratas. En un estudio limitado de la letalidad dominante en ratones no se registraron efectos en la fecundidad del macho. No se han comunicado investigaciones acerca de la fertilidad de las hembras ni estudios multigeneracionales.

2. Estudios en la especie humana

2.1 Efectos en el sistema nervioso

En muchos estudios se ha relacionado la exposición laboral al *n*-hexano con la frecuencia de la neuropatía periférica en la especie humana. Sin embargo, pocos de esos estudios informaban acerca de las concentraciones en el aire, los datos comunicados pueden ser inexactos y a menudo no está claro si esas concentraciones eran de hexano o de *n*-hexano. Además, la exposición industrial al *n*-hexano suele darse al utilizar productos a base de disolventes, de manera que los trabajadores están expuestos a una mezcla de compuestos volátiles (por ejemplo, acetato de etilo, metiletilcetona, tolueno, acetona y otros hidrocarburos alifáticos). Raramente se ha señalado la concentración en el aire de los otros disolventes presentes. En el presente examen sólo se han incluido los estudios que contenían algunos datos de las concentraciones en el aire.

Los resultados de la electrofisiología de los nervios periféricos pueden variar de manera considerable en función del tipo de técnica utilizada, la temperatura ambiente a la que se efectúan las mediciones, el segmento del nervio estudiado y la edad del individuo. Así pues, sin información sobre esos factores es difícil evaluar los estudios que se basan en la electrofisiología de los nervios periféricos.

Mediante el estudio de 93 casos de neuropatía se definieron las características clínicas de la producida por el *n*-hexano y se puso de manifiesto que existe una correlación clara entre las medidas electrofisiológicas y la gravedad de trastorno. Se encontró una relación entre el aumento de la gravedad y el de la exposición. Sin embargo, no fue posible establecer una relación definitiva a partir de los escasos detalles notificados sobre la exposición.

En los trabajadores del calzado expuestos a una concentración de 70 mg/m^3 (20 ppm) se encontraron signos subclínicos leves de neuropatía. El grado de anomalía electrofisiológica aumentaba con la duración de la exposición. Sin embargo, no se produjeron casos de neuropatía manifiesta, ni siquiera en trabajadores con una exposición de más de cinco años de duración.

Se observaron signos subjetivos y electrofisiológicos de neuropatía periférica subclínica en un grupo de trabajadores expuestos a 317 mg/m^3 (90 ppm). Sin embargo, esos efectos no se pueden atribuir exclusivamente a la exposición a esta concentración de *n*-hexano, puesto que probablemente se infravaloró la exposición anterior a disolventes y la autoselección de los trabajadores puede haber dado lugar a cierto sesgo. Además, se puede haber producido una exposición simultánea a la metiletilcetona, que, como se ha demostrado, aumenta los efectos neurotóxicos del *n*-hexano.

La exposición a una mezcla de disolventes con una concentración aproximada de *n*-hexano de 690 mg/m^3 (196 ppm) causó una reducción de la velocidad de conducción de los nervios periféricos, que se mantuvo tras disminuir la exposición de manera significativa. Se ha indicado asimismo que la causa de algunos de los cambios de potencial inducidos por estímulos somatosensoriales podría ser un efecto del *n*-hexano en el sistema nervioso central.

En un pequeño grupo de trabajadores expuestos a una concentración media de *n*-hexano en el aire de 208 mg/m^3 (59 ppm) se produjeron signos subjetivos y electrofisiológicos de una neuropatía subclínica leve. No se detectó neuropatía clínica manifiesta. En este estudio, la exposición a otros disolventes fue limitada y los estudios de conducción nerviosa se realizaron en condiciones definidas. Sin embargo, el pequeño número de individuos estudiados, la ausencia de historial de exposición y la escasa correspondencia entre los grupos de exposición y testigo limitan el valor de las conclusiones alcanzadas. No obstante, los resultados en general coinciden con los datos obtenidos en anteriores estudios de los que se informa más arriba. La exposición a 669 mg/m³ (190 ppm) durante períodos superiores a 8 h/día se asoció con la aparición de neuropatía periférica clínicamente manifiesta. Puede producirse una lenta recuperación parcial de la función nerviosa a lo largo de varios años. La exposición a concentraciones inferiores a 352 mg/m³ (100 ppm) no produjo neuropatía, pero aparecieron pruebas electrofisiológicas de efectos subclínicos.

En un pequeño grupo de trabajadores profesionalmente expuestos a niveles muy diversos de *n*-hexano en el aire se han descrito defectos en cuanto a la distinción de los colores y signos de maculopatía. La medición del potencial inducido por estímulos visuales y el electrorretinograma de esos individuos mostró anomalías en comparación con un grupo testigo de trabajadores no expuestos. También se ha informado de anomalías en el trazado del potencial causado por estímulos visuales en sujetos inhaladores de pegamento expuestos a *n*-hexano. Se ha indicado que puede producirse degeneración axonal en la vía óptica y que el *n*-hexano puede inducir un bloqueo de la conducción en el sistema nervioso central. También hay algunas pruebas de que existe cierta correlación entre los signos de maculopatía y los signos electrofisiológicos de neuropatía periférica. Se encontraron asimismo anomalías en el trazado electroencefalografico de algunos de los individuos estudiados.

2.2 *Otros efectos*

No se conoce ningún estudio sobre la fertilidad o los posibles efectos testiculares en los varones. Es muy escasa la información sobre la toxicidad aguda del *n*-hexano en la especie humana. La mayor parte de los estudios han consistido en la exposición a mezclas de disolventes. Los datos disponibles parecen indicar que el *n*-hexano tiene una toxicidad aguda baja.

Se han publicado muy pocos estudios sobre la irritación cutánea y ocular en voluntarios. El *n*-hexano es un agente ligeramente irritante que cuando entra en contacto durante un corto período con la piel del hombre causa un eritema pasajero. Se han descrito efectos más graves (eritema y vesículas) tras un contacto cutáneo oclusivo de cinco horas con *n*-hexano de tipo comercial. Se carece de datos suficientes para evaluar si el líquido puede causar en el hombre irritación ocular. No se observaron signos de irritación de los ojos en un estudio en que se expuso a un grupo de voluntarios a vapor de hexano con una concentración de 1760 mg/m^3 (500 ppm) durante 3-5 minutos. No se han comunicado casos de sensibilización cutánea en trabajadores expuestos y tampoco se ha observado en una prueba de maximización con *n*-hexano.

3. Efectos en el medio ambiente

El *n*-hexano es poco soluble en agua y muy volátil. Por consiguiente, la exposición de los organismos acuáticos es probablemente baja y pasajera, excepto en el caso de vertidos incontrolados en aguas de superficie. Los datos acerca de la toxicidad del *n*-hexano para los organismos acuáticos son escasos, variables, obtenidos en condiciones inapropiadas e insuficientes para evaluar del riesgo para el medio ambiente.

RECOMENDACIONES

1. Protección de la salud humana

La población general está expuesta a unas concentraciones de *n*-hexano a las que es improbable que corra algún riesgo. En relación con la salud en el trabajo, los niveles atmosféricos se deben mantener por debajo de los límites de exposición profesional recomendados, mediante el diseño de procesos de trabajo adecuados y por medio de controles técnicos, incluido el de la ventilación. En los espacios cerrados, en casos de emergencia y en determinadas actividades de mantenimiento se debe disponer de ropas protectoras adecuadas y protección de la respiración. Se recomienda el uso de respiradores con admisión de aire puro o respiradores autónomos con flujo continuo de oxígeno para concentraciones de *n*-hexano de hasta 8800 mg/m^3 (2500 ppm). En el caso de concentraciones entre 8800 mg/m^3 (2500 ppm) y 17 600 mg/m^3 (5000 ppm), el respirador debe llevar adaptada una protección facial completa. Aunque los guantes pueden impedir la penetración del *n*-hexano, las mezclas de éste con otros disolventes, como la metiletilcetona, pueden permitir al *n*-hexano pasar a través de los guantes y de otras prendas protectoras. Hay que tener en cuenta este factor cuando se utilicen mezclas de *n*-hexano.

2. Protección del medio ambiente

No es probable que el *n*-hexano represente un peligro para el medio ambiente, excepto en el caso de derrames o vertidos importantes, que podrían provocar efectos locales pasajeros.

NUEVAS INVESTIGACIONES

a) Se debería hacer un estudio sobre los índices de la función testicular en uno o varios grupos de trabajadores expuestos para establecer si alguno o todos los efectos cuya presencia se ha descrito en los testículos de los animales se manifiestan también en el hombre.

b) Conviene seguir investigando *in vivo* los efectos genotóxicos del *n*-hexano, a fin de complementar la limitada información que se posee sobre estos efectos *in vitro*.

c) Para establecer la toxicidad del *n*-hexano administrado por vía oral es necesario realizar un estudio de dosis repetidas. Es preciso hacer esto para determinar el nivel sin efecto observado, a fin de definir una ingesta diaria admisible (IDA).

d) No está claro el mecanismo de la neurotoxicidad a nivel molecular. Su conocimiento contribuirá directamente a la validez de la evaluación del riesgo. Se necesitar estudios *in vivo* e *in vitro* para seguir investigando y aclarar esos mecanismos.

e) Los estudios de teratogenia disponibles no bastan para evaluar el riesgo. Conviene realizar estudios que proporcionen datos utilizables.

f) No se conoce la relación dosis-respuesta en cuanto a los efectos neurotóxicos del *n*-hexano en la especie humana, debido a que los datos de exposición son incompletos o no fidedignos. Además, aunque se ha demostrado ampliamente la neurotoxicidad periférica del *n*-hexano, los efectos en el sistema nervioso central sólo se han examinado de forma limitada. Deben realizarse más investigaciones epidemiológicas, como por ejemplo estudios prospectivos de seguimiento, para subsanar la escasez de datos de las anteriores investigaciones.